PROEM

   THE king stood in his hall of offering,
On either hand the white-robed Brahmans ranged
Muttered their mantras, feeding still the fire
Which roared upon the midmost altar. There
From scented woods flickered bright tongues of flaunt
Hissing and curling as they licked the gifts
Of ghee and spices and the Soma juice,
The joy of Indra. Round about the pile
A slow, thick, scarlet streamlet smoked and ran,
Sucked by the sand, but ever rolling down.
The blood of bleating victims. One such lay,
A spotted goat, long-horned, its head bound back
With munja grass; at its stretched throat the knife
Pressed by a priest, who murmured, 'This, dread gods
Of many yajnas, cometh as the crown
From Bimbasâra; take ye joy to see
The spirted blood, and pleasure in the scent
Of rich flesh roasting 'mid the fragrant flames;
Let the king's sins be laid upon this goat,
And let the fire consume them burning it,
For now I strike.'
But Buddha softly said,
'Let him not strike, great king!' and therewith loosed
The victim's bonds, none staying him, so great
 His presence was. Then, craving leave, he spake
 Of life, which all can take but none can give,
Life, which all creatures love and strive to keep,
Wonderful, dear, and pleasant unto each,
Even to the meanest; yea, a boon to all
Where pity is, for pity nukes the world
Soft to the weak and noble for the strong.
Unto the dumb lips of the flock he lent
Sad, pleading words, showing how man, who prays

For mercy to the gods, is merciless.
Being as god to those; albeit all life
Is linked and kin, and what we slay have given
Meek tribute of their milk and wool, and set
Fast trust upon the hands which murder them.
Also he spake of what the holy books
Do surely teach, how that at death some sink
To bird and beast, and these rise up to man
In wanderings of the spark which grows purged flame.
So were the sacrifice new sin, if so
The fated passage of a soul be stayed.
Nor spake he, shall one wash his spirit clean
By blood; nor gladden gods, being good, with blood
Nor bribe them, being evil; nay, nor lay
Upon the brow of innocent bound beasts
One hair's weight of that answer all must give
For all things done amiss or wrongfully,
Alone, each for himself, reckoning with that
The fixed arithmic of the universe,
Which meteth good for good and ill for ill,
Men are for measure, unto deeds, words, thoughts;
Watchful, aware, implacable, unmoved;
Making all futures fruits of all the pasts.
Thus spake he, breathing words so piteous
With such high lordliness of ruth and right,
The priests drew back their garments o'er the hand
Crimsoned with slaughter, and the king came near.
Standing with clasped palms reverencing Buddha;
While still our Lord went on, teaching how fair
This earth were if all living things be linked
In friendliness and common use of foods.
Bloodless and pure; the golden grain, bright fruits.
Sweet herbs which grow for all, the waters wan,
Sufficient drinks and meats. Which when these heard,
The might of gentleness so conquered them,
The priests themselves scattered their altar-flames
And flung away the steel of sacrifice;
And Through the land next day passed a decree
Proclaimed by criers, and in this wise graved
On rock and column: 'Thus the king's will is:
There hath been slaughter for the sacrifice
And slaying for the meat, but henceforth none
Shall spill the blood of life nor taste of flesh,
Seeing that knowledge grows, and life is one,

The Perfect Way in Diet

A treatise advocating a return to the natural and ancient food of our race

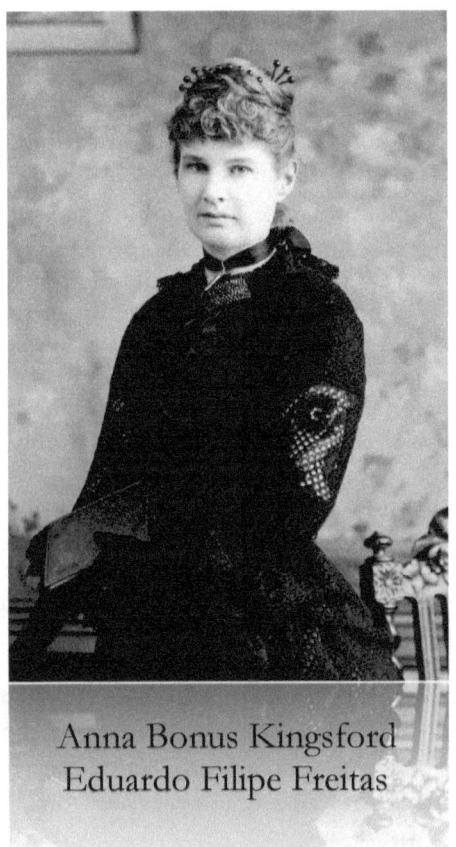

Anna Bonus Kingsford
Eduardo Filipe Freitas

Copyright © 2018 Eduardo Filipe Freitas
All rights reserved.
eduardofilipef@gmail.com
+351913088176

ISBN: 1985666448
ISBN-13: 978-1985666443

PREFACE

The following treatise is a translation, revised and enlarged, of my *'These pour le Doctorat'* which, under the title *'De l'Alimentation Végétale chez l'Homme,'* I presented in the month of July, 1880, at the *Faculté de Médicine of Paris* on completing my medical studies and taking my degree.

The original thesis was published in Paris in the French language, and subsequently translated into German and issued with illustrative notes and other additions by Dr. A. Aderholdt Encouraged by the success obtained by these two editions, and by the favourable notices they elicited from various foreign scientific and popular critics, I offer the present work to English readers, confident of a kindly welcome from the friends of the reform I advocate, and hopeful of a serious and intelligent hearing from those who as yet are strangers to the merits of that reform.

The French and German editions of this treatise include an Appendix, containing short notices and citations from the works of the chief exponents and exemplars of the Pythagorean system of diet. In the present volume this Appendix is suppressed in favour of a forthcoming 'Catena of Authorities Denunciatory or Depreciatory of the Practice of Flesh-Eating,' by a 'Graduate of Cambridge'; an excellent and ample compendium to which the reader is referred.

That I have dwelt chiefly on the aspects, physical and social, of my subject, and touched but lightly on those moral and philosophical, is not, assuredly, because I regard these last as of lesser importance, but because their abstruse and recondite nature renders them unsuitable to a work intended for general reading.

Finally, if any into whose hands this book may fall, should be inclined to think me over-enthusiastic, or to stigmatise my views as 'Utopian,' I would ask him seriously to consider whether 'Utopia' be not indeed within the realisation of all who can imagine and love it, and whether, without enthusiasm, any great cause was ever yet won for our race. Man is the master of the world, and may make it what he will. Into his hands it is delivered with all its mighty possibilities for good or evil, for happiness or misery. Following the monitions and devices of the sub-human, he may make of it – what indeed for some gentle and tender souls it has already become – a very hell; working with God and Nature, he may reconvert it into Paradise.

ANNA KINGSFORD, M.D.
II CHAPEL STREET, PARK LANE,
Michaelmas, 1881.

And mercy cometh to the merciful.'
So ran the edict, and from those days forth
Sweet peace hath spread between all living kind,
Man and the beasts which serve him, and the birds,
On all those banks of Ganga where our Lord
Taught with his saintly pity and soft speech. *(1)*

FOOTNOTES

(xii:1) The Light of Asia; being the Life and Teaching of Gautama, Founder of Buddhism. By Edwin Arnold.

1. ANATOMY AND PHYSIOLOGY

BY what habits and mode of life has humanity in the past attained its highest development, and what is the method which modern science and philosophy indicate to us as that best adapted to perfect our kind?

In order to resolve this vast and important inquiry, it will be necessary, in the first place, to refer to natural history, and seek in the study of the comparative anatomy of men and other animals for information regarding the primitive habits of mankind, and the mode of living which is indicated by their exterior conformation and by the structure of their organs. In short, we must inquire whether the human race is naturally carnivorous, herbivorous, omnivorous, or frugivorous. Without accepting definitively the theories of Lamarck, Darwin, and Haeckel, I think we may adopt, without fear of any serious objection, the classification of Linnaeus, which is generally admitted by scientists. This classification distinguishes, under the name of Primates, the highest order in the class of mammiferous animals, and at its head is placed the human family and that of the anthropoid apes. This last contains two species, one of which, from an anatomical and physiological point of view, resembles man very closely; I mean the apes of the Old World, among which we find the orang-outan (wild man), the gorilla, and the chimpanzee. The orang belongs to the tribe of the Simiadae, the gorilla and the chimpanzee to the Troglodytes.

We will examine as rapidly and shortly as possible the characters which attach these creatures to man, and those which separate them, as well as man, from certain other orders or genera. Next we shall inquire what mode of alimentation is proper to the animals most resembling the human family, and thus we shall be enabled to judge what ought to be, consistently with natural laws, the habits and diet of the latter. We will begin our task by an examination of the superior part of the skeleton, the cranium, and the organs it contains.

The most superficial observation enables us to recognise on the one hand the resemblance which exists between the general conformation of the skull of man and that of the ape, and on the other hand the differences which establish a line of separation more or less marked between the human cranium and that belonging to other mammalia of no matter what order or species. Passing by these familiar and superficial features of morphology, we will devote ourselves to the study of those which present a more scientific and less common interest.

The noblest and most important apparatus of the animal economy is without doubt the nervous system, which, dominating the functions of all the organs, presides over the harmony of their operations, regulates the work of all other systems and tissues, repairs their lesions, maintains their integrity, and is, as it were, preserver and law-giver of the bodily kingdom. The animal in which this system, and above all, the dominant part of this system, that is to say the brain, appears to resemble the human type most closely, will therefore possess, a Priori, the right to be considered the most man-like among the lower races. Moreover, it is to the perfection, more or less accentuated, of the nervous system, and in particular to that of its ganglionic centres – that is, to the more or less perfect aggregation and complete composition of the parts which constitute this system – that are due principally, we might almost say exclusively, the degree of elevation of any given being in the animal scale, and the characters which separate it more or less distinctly from the vegetable kingdom. Now it is in man that we find the supreme degree of this aggregation and ganglionic development, and the animal which most closely imitates him in this respect is the orang-outan. The height of the brain in the orang is greater than in the chimpanzee, the frontal lobe is more developed, the occipital smaller, the temporal more horizontal and less flattened – characteristics which well agree with the exterior aspect of the simians. Besides, the brain convolutions, which are very rudimentary in the rodents and edentates, less simple in the carnassiers, and still less so in the ruminants and solipedes, attain their greatest development in the apes, and particularly in the orang. The disposition of the cerebral mass in the carnivorous mammals, which has been well studied by Leuret, shows only six convolutions, varying in regularity and simplicity according to the species, but remaining in all cases parallel to each other and antero-posterior in direction. These convolutions have been described by Professor Sappey under the name of constant or primitive convolutions. It is not until we reach the elephant, the lemur, and particularly the ape-group, that we find certain new convolutions, or 'folds of perfectionment' remarkable by their volume and by their perpendicular direction to the primitive convolutions. 'Add,' says M. Sappey, 'to the antero-posterior convolutions of the carnivora and other inferior mammals, two or three convolutions cutting them perpendicularly in the middle, and the disposition proper to the highest mammals, particularly man and the ape, will be realised.'

Now in the brain of the orang we not only find the antero-posterior convolutions lengthened, curved, and anastomosed after the human type, but it is also in the encephalon of the same animal that those additional convolutions or 'folds of perfectionment' noticed by Professor Sappey appear the roost distinctly, and offer consequently the completest analogy with the disposition of the cerebral organ in man. We are thus authorised to conclude, with Professor Mivart, (1) that the difference between the brain of the orang and that of the human subject is one not of kind, but of degree. The writings of the late Professor Broca, whose careful studies in anthropology give special weight to his statements, confirm this opinion, and assert that the brain of the archencephalous animals – hominidae of Owen – differs so little from that of the superior gyrencephalae that the only distinctive characters observable in the latter are altogether secondary in importance. 'But,' says the professor, 'these characters are not real in their nature, and even if they were, even if the cerebral hemispheres of the apes contained neither the ancyroid cavity nor the small hippocampus of man, even if we should find their cerebrum not entirely covering the cerebellum, these differences would be but slight, almost accessory, and less important than those which we meet with among animals belonging to the same order, so that they must be held altogether insufficient for the establishment of two sub-classes.'

Having thus briefly traced the points of resemblance between the human and the simian brain, and their common divergence from the type presented by other and lower races, we pass to the examination of the buccal cavity, which ought to furnish us with valuable indications respecting the mode of life of the subject under observation.

In the anthropoid animals the mouth is disposed according to the human type. The lateral sacks, known as cheek-pouches, are absent in this species; the two excretory canals of the sub-maxillary glands (Wharton's ducts) open singly on the sides of the fraenum of the tongue; the tongue itself resembles that of man; in the orang the circumvallate papillae present the V-shaped disposition of the human type, their arrangement slightly differing in the chimpanzee and assuming the form of a T. The dental morphology and formula of the apes of the old world (catarrhines) are identical with those of man; their cuspids are, however, longer, especially in the males, and the wisdom teeth appear at an earlier age than in the human subject The apes of the New World (platyrrhines) differ from man by the absence of one molar in each half-jaw, the place of this tooth being occupied by an extra bicuspid. The surface of the molar teeth in the human subject is characterised by the presence of an irregular ramified depression dividing it into four or five distinct tubercules. The same formation is met with in the orang, the chimpanzee, and the gorilla, as also is the superficial disposition of the enamel, which substance, in the herbivorous races, is quite otherwise distributed. Among the latter, pachydermata, ruminants (which have no incisors in the upper jaw), and rodents, the molar teeth are composed of alternate layers of dentine, enamel, and cement, which penetrate into the interior of the tooth, so that a transverse section of it, instead of presenting an homogeneous substance surrounded by a simple enamel stratum, as in man and the quadrumana, exhibits several undulating composite folds.. the dentine of which, being much less durable than the enamel, wears down rapidly, and the tooth thus acquires a rough unequal surface fitted to triturate the woody substances which form pan of the alimentation of these animals. On the other hand, the carnassiers possess organs of mastication, which, according to Küss, are hardly properly called teeth, but rather spike-like instruments destined to tear in fragments the meat on which they feed. Their incisives, six instead of four in number in each jaw, are small, pointed, and uneven; the surface of the molar teeth exhibits the appearance of a saw, and there usually exists but one on each side, the last bicuspid or carnassial tooth being especially characteristic. This tooth, well developed in the tiger kind, is composed of three sharp strong uneven prominences, placed one behind the other and connected by jutting ridges, the anterior prominence being doubled by an accessory spine. Nothing of this sort is observable in man or in the races which stand nearest to him. By the side of the exclusively predatory mammals we place the omnivorous types, such as the Alpine bear, the North American bear (ursus arctos), the wild boar, and the hog (sus scrofa, sus tibetanus, and sus ibericus). In the bear the surface of the molars is flattened, but the incisives number six as in the true carnivora, although they are blunter and less accentuated than the corresponding teeth of the latter. The cuspids are very long and curved, and between them and the bicuspids a remarkable interval generally exists. This character of dentition resembles the carnivorous rather than the herbivorous type, and, except that the enamel is superficially placed upon the cheek teeth, has nothing in common with the human and frugivorous morphology. The incisive teeth of the wild boar and the hog are elongated, and project forward in the direction of the axe of the maxillary bone; the cuspids, particularly those of the superior jaw, assume a special character, and develop themselves in the shape of tusks; in the lower jaw these teeth projecting outwards cross the direction of the upper pair. The same interval between the cuspids and the premolars, which we noted in the bear, exists also in the boar and pig species.

Let us now pass to an examination of the zygomatic arch and temporal region in the various orders of the mammalia. This region is important to our subject, because its disposition and aspect serve to indicate the kind of food proper to the animal It is to be remarked that in man and in the apes the zygomatic arch is comparatively frail, slightly curved so as to present an upper concave surface, and that the tempora and masseter muscles are but little developed; while in the ruminants, although the temporal muscle does not attain any important dimensions, the masseter on the contrary manifests considerable development, and. passing beyond the zygomatic arch, attaches itself to nearly the whole of the lateral surface of the superior maxillary. Moreover the inferior jaw of these latter animals possesses a lateral movement, which is quite characteristic, and to produce it the condyles are flattened and enabled to slide sideways in their cavity of reception. Another type of condyle is that of the rodents, which exhibits an increased diameter in the antero-posterior sense, and has a glenoid cavity similarly hollowed.

But it is pre-eminently among the carnivorous quadrupeds that we meet with the most striking variation from the human type in respect to the characters of the temporal arch. The zygomatic arch in the flesh-eating animals is extremely large, and is increased in strength by its decided curve, the direction of which is the reverse of that which we have noted in the frugivora; for the concavity is inferior in position and the upper surface is strongly convex, the curve increasing with the ferocity of the species. The dimensions, as well as the peculiar form, of this bone, and its outward projection from the skull, give strength precisely in the direction most required, and augment enormously the tearing power. Besides, the masseter and temporal muscles are strongly developed, the thickness of the latter entirely filling the large space between the zygomatic process and the temporal bone; while in height it attains the upper limit of the skull On the other hand the internal and external pterygoidan muscles are very small, because these quadrupeds possess no lateral mobility of the jaw. This movement indeed is rendered impossible by the disposition of the glenoid cavity, the great depth of which prevents any change of position other than perpendicular opening and shutting. The omnivora differ but very slightly from the carnassiers in these respects; and it is only among the apes and above all the simians and troglodytes that we find a disposition and aspect of this articulation and muscular region perfectly analogous to those observable in man.

The classification which we have thus seen indicated in regard to the brain, the buccal cavity, the teeth and the temporo-maxillary articulation, will be confirmed by a study of the digestive canal.

The human stomach is simple, consisting, that is, of a single receptacle, as is that of all the primates. Professor Broca kindly allowed me to see in his anthropological laboratory, some drawings and anatomical preparations which demonstrated in a most striking manner the identity of configuration which exists between the digestive apparatus of man and that of the superior apes. Indeed it is at first sight barely possible to distinguish between the two, though a close comparison will show the human stomach to be smaller than that of the ape. As for the intestine, the anthropoids do not differ from man in this respect; their caecum, deprived of mesentery, is fixed in the right iliac fossa by the peritoneum, the vermiform appendix exists in all animals of the tribe, and the length of the entire tract accords with the human type. The liver of the orang (and gibbon) is as simple as that of man; in the chimpanzee this organ seems less developed, for its 'lobule of Spigel' is smaller and the fissure of the inferior vena cava is reduced to a mere depression. We may note that with regard to the liver, as in some other respects, the anthropoids differ considerably from the last three families of the primates, and do not differ in any sensible degree from man. The gall-bladder is always present in all the primates; among other mammals it is absent in the cetacea, sloths, rhinoceri, elephants, camels, horses, and tapirs. The peritoneum and the omenta of the orang are almost identical in arrangement with the same membranes in man, and we must remember that the peritoneal folds have considerable importance, for their connexions and complicated dispositions are the consequence of certain alterations of position undergone by the abdominal viscera during embryonic evolution. In one small detail the chimpanzee differs from man in this respect; the omentum of the former is attached to the upper part of the ascending colon for a very limited distance. In this animal, as in the gorilla and the orang, the ascending colon, and the superior part of the caecum are fixed by the peritoneum to the side of the vertebral column in the came manner as in the human subject (1). The stomach of the carnivorous quadrupeds differs from the same organ in man in regard not only to its relative dimensions, but to its form. Instead of being subdivided, as in the frugivorous races, into cardiac and pyloric portions, the carnivorous stomach is formed like a simple bag, elongated slightly in a transversal sense, and is throughout of the same capacity. The length of the digestive canal, compared with that of the whole body, varies in the carnivorous races from three to six for one:, while in the apes and in man the proportion is from seven to ten for one, The liver of the carnivora presents, in respect of general conformation, a much more complicated division than the human organ, being composed of six distinct lobes or parts. There is usually no caecum; in those instances in which it exists it is always rudimentary.

On the other hand, the stomach of the herb-eaters, especially that of the ruminants, possesses a very complicated form, and even when a comparatively simple organ exists, as in the horse, the caecum and colon present an advanced development which seems calculated to compensate for the want of complexity presented by the stomach. We find in the ruminants four distinct receptacles – the rumen or paunch, the reticulum, the psalterium or many-plies, and the abomasum or rennet; and the length of the digestive canal, compared with that of the whole body, varies from twelve to twenty-seven for one. Not to omit the omnivorous quadrupeds, we will take the hog as a fair specimen of the class. In this animal we find the cardiac fundus dilated into a pouch, unlike the human type while two parallel folds conduct from the oesophagus to the pylorus.

The celebrated experiments of Dr. Beaumont upon Alex's Saint Martin have demonstrated that the peristaltic movements of the human stomach take place in the sense of a complete revolution; in other words, that portion of the alimentary mass which at any given moment occupies the greater curvature, moves to the right towards the pylorus, while that portion of the mass which occupies the lesser curvature moves to the left towards the cardiac. There is then a continuous peristaltic movement on the side of the greater curvature, and an anti-peristaltic movement on the side of the lesser curvature.

Now it appears to be established that it is thus the digestive movements of the stomach are produced in herborous animals, and without doubt it is thus also that they take place in mammals of the order to which man himself belongs; but in the carnivora there exists only a simple action to-and-fro from left to right and from right to left. (1) It does not appear that any opportunity has arisen of observing these movements in omnivorous animals, but analogy leads to the belief that no difference in this respect would be found between the latter and the .true carnassiers.

With regard to the comparative analysis of the different digestive juices of the economy, it is advisable to make a few comments:

1. The opportunities which present themselves for the study of their composition in the physiological, that is, in the healthy state, in the human subject, are exceedingly rare; and the same may be said in the case of other animals; for the preliminary operations necessary for the creation of fistula, etc., complicate so greatly the conditions under which these juices are obtained, that it is hardly possible to regard as conclusive the results which their analysis affords. It is highly probable that in the greater number of such cases, the secretions are altered some time before the operator can succeed in isolating the constituent elements.

2. The secretions of the economy vary with the nature of the alimentation, and it seems probable that were it possible to compare the digestive juices of a person habitually kreophagist with those of another habitually vegetarian, a chemical difference would be distinctly noticeable. It is in fact well known that the functions and secretions of the organism accommodate themselves with more or less ease and rapidity to the habits of life and food of the individual. Thus, in the carnivorous animal, the quantity of saliva produced during a repast is proportionately much less than in the herb-feeder, and the kreophagist man secretes relatively but little. But the same man, it appears, after becoming vegetarian, experiences a notable increase in the secretion of his salivary glands, which thus adapt their function to the necessities of his new regimen; and although it is unfortunate that we cannot refer to any comparative analysis in such cases, one would logically be brought to suppose that the chemical properties of the digestive juices would, as readily as the mechanical process, adapt themselves to new conditions of subsistence.

But notwithstanding these restrictive remarks, it appears, according to Bernard, Lent, and others, that the human saliva, even in the ordinary kreophagist conditions, bears a stronger resemblance to that of the herbivorous than to that of the carnivorous animals, for like the former it possesses the power of saccharification, which has not been discovered in the corresponding secretion of any of the carnivora, the action assigned to the saliva in these latter bearing exclusive relation to the mechanics of mastication and deglutition. It has also been demonstrated by the studies of Frerichs and Gorup-Besanez (1) that the human bile presents the same composition as that of the herbivora.

In terminating this portion of our work, we may just glance at the difference which exists with regard to the disposition and extent of the sudoriparous glands between the carnassiers on the one hand and the anthropoids and herbivora on the other, the alimentation of these last giving rise naturally to the formation of an excess of heat, and demanding therefore a more extensive apparatus for its elimination. Man in this respect also resembles the fruit and herb eaters.

If we have consecrated to this sketch of comparative anatomy and physiology a paragraph which may seem a little wearisome in detail, it is because it appears necessary to combat certain erroneous impressions affecting the structure of man which obtain credence, not only in the vulgar world, but even among otherwise instructed persons. How many times, for instance, have we not heard people speak with all the authority of conviction about the 'canine teeth' and 'simple stomach' of man, as certain evidence of his natural adaptation for a flesh diet! At least we have demonstrated one fact; that if such arguments are valid, they apply with even greater force to the anthropoid apes – whose 'canine' teeth are much longer and more powerful than those of man – and the scientists must make haste therefore to announce a rectification of their present division of the Animal Kingdom in order to class with the carnivora and their proximate species, all those animals which now make up the order of Primates. And yet, with the solitary exception of man, there is not one of these last which does not in a natural condition absolutely refuse to feed on flesh! (1) M. Pouchet observes (2) that all the details of the digestive apparatus in man, as well as his dentition, constitute 'so many proofs of his frugivorous origin' – an opinion shared by Professor Owen, who remarks that the anthropoids and all the quadrumana derive their alimentation from fruits, grains, and other succulent and nutritive vegetable substances, and that the strict analogy which exists between the structure of these animals and that of man clearly demonstrates his frugivorous nature. This is also the view taken by Cuvier, (3) Linnaeus, Professor Lawrence, (4) Charles Bell, (5) Gassendi, Flourens, and a great number of other eminent writers. The last named scientist gives expression to his views after the following manner:

– 'Man is neither carnivorous nor herbivorous. He has neither the teeth of the cud-chewers, nor their four stomachs, nor their intestines. If we consider these organs in man, we must conclude him to be by nature and origin frugivorous, as is the ape.'

It may possibly be objected that since, according to natural structure and propensities, man is a fruit and seed eater, he ought not to partake of those leguminous plants and roots which belong rather to the dietary of the herb-eaters, whose organisation we have shown to differ in so many details from that of man. It may be urged that trouble is wasted in proving to what order man belongs by nature, since with him, alone of all animals, Art has superseded Nature, and has enabled him by means of fire, condiments, and disguise, to eat and digest without disgust, and even with relish, the food of the tiger, the wolf, and the hyena.

2. COOKERY

Such objections are not without an air of reason; and I shall meet them first by the frank statement that the most excellent and proper aliments of which our race can make use consist of tree-fruits and seeds, *(1)* and not of the plants themselves, whether foliage or roots. But through a combination of natural and artificial causes, this best mode of subsistence has become impossible to the majority of persons in certain parts of the globe, and it seems therefore wise and consistent that they should increase the variety and range of their food by recourse to cookery. Fire can, however, be only used legitimately by man for the preparation of those vegetables, herbaceous plants, roots, and hard fruits, which he cannot properly masticate when raw, and for the digestion of which, in that condition, the anatomy and physiology of his system are not adapted. The true frugivora, of which he is a member, do not refuse to eat produce of this kind when thus prepared, even in countries where fruits are procurable; and it is well known that in the *Jardin des Plantes* (Paris) and other menageries, the daily rations of the monkeys are composed of bread, cooked potatoes, salad, and apples – a dietary derived, therefore, from cereals, tubers, herbs, and fruit. Such substances as these are not distasteful to frugivorous feeders; on the contrary, their odours and their aspect are alike inviting to the palate, and even in their unprepared state they are agreeable to sight, smell, and idea. But for man, the choice between Nature and Art, between the garden and the slaughter-house, involves far larger issues and far deeper-reaching considerations than can be held to touch the mere anthropoid. The culture, harvesting, and preparation of all vegetable produce are alike in harmony with the interests of morality, of individual and of public health, of social and private economy, and of that love of beauty, virtue, and consistent philosophy which dominates the nature of all gentle and civilised humanity. Each one of these interests, on the contrary, is wounded, and that violently, as I am about to show, by the abuse of the art of cookery in the hands of the man who degrades himself by its means to the level of the beast of prey.

Thus we have shown that mankind are naturally frugivorous; and we know that they can also become both omnivorous and carnivorous. Let us proceed to inquire therefore whether, from any point of view, such transformations of their nature are attended with advantage to the race or individual.

FOOTNOTES

(10:1) Broca, '*L'ordre des Primates*.' Bulletins de la Société d'Antroplogie, vol. iv.
(11:1) Béclard and Schults.
(13:1) Etudes sur des Suppliciés.
(14:1) Broca Mivart, Owen, etc.
(14:2) Pluralité de la race humaine, p. 39.
(14:3) Règne animal.
(14: 4) Lectures on Physiology.
(14:5) Diseases of the Teeth.
(15:1) And these uncooked.

3. PHYSICAL FORCE

Now the idea that attributes to man an organisation which he does not possess is not more common than is another belief equally false; I mean the opinion that flesh-food contains the elements of physical force, and that to be strong, robust, and endowed with muscular energy, it is necessary to partake largely of animal food. This belief, like the former, finds partisans not only among the general public, but in the world of medical teachers and practitioners, who, for the most part, have adopted the opinions and faith of the vulgar upon the strength, not of scientific examination, but of accepted custom. Nevertheless, we daily see in our fields and our streets ample evidence that the strongest, the usefullest, and the most capable workers among the animals are precisely those which never taste flesh-meat Their force and their endurance are invincible, and surpass beyond comparison that of their beef-fed masters. All the labour of the world is performed by the herbivora – horses, oxen, mules, elephants, camels; by these our fields are ploughed, our cities built, our battles fought, our journeys accomplished, and to these is man largely indebted for the existence of civilisation, commerce, and national wealth. No carnivorous animal can boast the enormous power of the herb-fed rhinoceros, who breaks with scarce an effort trunks of trees, and grinds whole branches to powder like so many wisps of hay; no carnassier exhibits the endurance and stay of the horse, who toils with hardly any rest from morning to night under the weight of immense burdens, and whose strength has passed into a proverb. Du Chaillu reports that he saw a gorilla, nourished with simple fruits and nuts, break in his hands, with no apparent effort, the gun accidentally dropped by one of his pursuers; and an eminent naturalist, Dr. Duncan, F.R.S., assures us that this animal in his native wilds is more than a match for the African lion.

The buffalo, the bison, the hippopotamus, the bull, the zebra, the stag, are types of physical power and vast bulk, or of splendid development of limb, built up, not mediately from the flesh and blood of fellow organisms, but from the original sources of strength itself – the wild plants and fruit and herb of the field

The carnivora indeed possess one salient and terrible quality, ferocity, allied to thirst for blood; but power, endurance, courage, and intelligent capacity for toil, belong to those animals who alone, since the world had a history, have been associated with the fortunes, the conquests, and the achievements of men.

And here we will take occasion to observe that the nations who have left to us the most superb monument, the most glorious records, the profoundest and the purest thought, were not kreophagist nations. The opening chapters of the Hebrew book of Genesis, the origin of which is Egyptian, plainly declare what tradition this great people – mother of all the arts and sciences in the world – held with regard to the nature of man, and of his food in the perfect state. And we are informed by investigators of antiquarian records that the habits and primitive religion of ancient Egypt, and of Ethiopia – perhaps the oldest of all human colonies – absolutely forbade the use of animal meats. *(1)*

FOOTNOTES

(18:1) See Samuel Sharpe's *History of Egypt*.

4. NATIONAL HABITS

What would our athletes of to-day say to the regimen of the Grecian wrestlers and pugilists of antiquity, whose degenerated shadows they are? In the gymnasia or palestrae, academies of the athletic profession, where persons destined to the acquirement of the art were trained from early youth, the masters subjected their neophytes to those methods which they judged the most efficacious for the production and augmentation of physical strength and power of resistance to fatigue. And one of the means employed for accomplishing this object was the enforcement of a very severe and frugal dietary, composed only of figs, nuts, cheese, and maize bread, without wine. *(2)* In the palmy days of Greece and Rome, before intemperance and licentious living had robbed those kingdoms of their glory and greatness, their sons, who were not only soldiers but heroes, subsisted on simple vegetable food, rye meal, fruits, and milk. The chief food of the Roman gladiator was barley cakes and oil; and this diet, Hippocrates says, is eminently fitted to give muscular strength and endurance. The daily rations of the Roman soldier were one pound of barley, three ounces of oil, and a pint of thin wine. It was no regimen of flesh that inspired the magnificent courage of the Spartan patriots who defended the defiles of Thermopylae, or that filled with indomitable valour and enthusiasm the conquerors of Salamis and Marathon. And even in these days it must not be forgotten that the kreophagist nations constitute little more than a quarter of the human race, and it is precisely among this fourth part of mankind that the greatest amount of misery, crime, and disease is found.

The Hindoos are divided into several castes or distinct orders, a division which dates from the remotest antiquity. Of these orders the highest, which is that of the Brahmins, attributes its origin to the head of the Creator, while the lowest is figured as issuing from his feet. The three superior castes, Brahmins, Kshattriyas, and Vaisyas, are by their religious precepts forbidden the use of animal meats; for the practice of kreophagy is, in the Hindoo mind, associated with ideas of pollution and degradation, and a pure vegetable diet is regarded as the first essential of sanctity. And we must remember that this venerable and important race possesses a cultus, a literature, and a religious system which many authors deem to be of higher antiquity than those even of Egypt; and that consequently the national laws of Hindostan reflect the true image of the world's early instincts, and of the primitive manners of the first civilised communities, before the advent of that vital and moral decline which, in later ages, luxury imported into the habits of our great commercial centres.

The larger part of the population of China and Japan consists of Buddhists, whose traditions are analogous to those of the Brahmins. Buddha Sakyamouni, the Christ of their faith, absolutely condemned the use of flesh-food among the elect; and the pious Buddhist not only avoids killing animals, but believes he performs a meritorious act in succouring them or in showing them kindness. The murder of a cow is punished by scourging, and imprisonment during two months; a repetition of the offence entails banishment. Conceive the horror which would be felt by a Brahmin or Buddhist educated in such sentiments and accustomed to such modes of thought as these, were he to be brought face to face with the spectacles which every moment confront us in our Christian streets and markets; imagine his astonishment at the phenomenon presented by a religion whose principal holy days are celebrated by the massacre of untold multitudes of beasts and birds of every kind, and by bloody repasts in which the most fervent devotees and the priests themselves take eager part!

The following brief résumé of facts collected from many various sources will enable the reader to see at a glance how wide a range of climate and of race the vegetarian question embraces, and how high under this regimen has been and is the standard of human health and physical strength.

EGYPT. – Edwin de Leon, in a work entitled *'The Khedive's Egypt,'* 1877, writing of the Egyptian fellah or peasant proprietor, says 'His living expenses are miraculously small Bread and vegetables are his food, Nile water his drink.' 'In Egypt,' says another writer, 'the diet of the peasantry and labouring people is much the same as in China. They use fish as a kind of relish or condiment, but their nourishment is derived from vegetable substances. Their food chiefly consists of coarse bread made of wheat, millet, or maize, together with cucumbers, melons, gourds, onions, leeks, beans, chickpease, lupins, lentils, dates, etc. Most of these vegetables they eat in a raw state." *(1)*

'It is indeed surprising to observe how simple and poor is the diet of the Egyptian peasantry, and yet how robust and healthy most of them are, and how severe is the labour they undergo. The boatmen of the Nile are mostly strong, muscular men, rowing, poling, and towing continually; but very cheerful, and often the most so when most occupied, for then they amuse themselves by singing.' *(2)*

'The Egyptian cultivators of the soil, who live on coarse wheaten bread, Indian bread, lentils, and other productions of the vegetable kingdom, are among the finest people I have ever seen.' *(3)*

INDIA. – 'From the earliest period the most general food in India has been rice, which is still the most common food of nearly all the hottest countries in Asia. It is not, however, so much used in the south of Hindostan as formerly, and has been replaced by another grain called rági.' *(4)*

'The principal food of the people of Hindostan is wheat, and in the Deckan, jowár and bájra; rice, as a general article of subsistence, is confined to Bengal and part of Behár, with the low country along the sea all round the coast of the peninsula. In most parts of India it is a luxury. In the southern part of the tableland of the Deckan, the body of the people live on a small and poor grain called rági . . . Pulse, roots, and fruits are also largely eaten.' *(5)*

In Sir John Sinclair's time (1818), before modern facilities had obviated the necessity of employing pedestrian messengers, the Pattamar Hindoos, occupied in carrying letters and despatches by land, performed journeys almost incredible in the time allotted. Thus from Calcutta to Bombay twenty-five days were allowed (about sixty-two miles a day), from Madras to Bombay, eighteen days; from Surat to Bombay, three days and a half. 'These men,' says Sir John, 'are generally tall, being from five feet ten inches to six feet high. They subsist on a little boiled rice.'

MEXICO.– 'The usual food of the labouring classes, throughout such states as I visited, is the thin cake of crushed maize, which I have described under the name of tortilla; and it is remarkable that, notwithstanding the great abundance of cattle in many places, the traveller can rarely obtain meat in the little huts which he finds on his road. Chilis are eaten abundantly with the tortillas, being stewed in a kind of sauce, into which the cakes are dipped.' *(1)*

'The Indians of new Spain generally attain to a pretty advanced age . . . They are accustomed to uniform nourishment of an almost entirely vegetable nature, that of their maize and cereal gramma.' *(2)*

CHILI. – 'It is usual for the copper-miners of Central Chili to carry loads of ore of two hundred pounds weight up eighty perpendicular yards twelve times a day. When they reach the mouth of the pit they are in a state of apparent fearful exhaustion, yet, after briefly resting, they descend again. Their diet is entirely vegetable: breakfast of figs and small loaves of bread; dinner, boiled beans; supper, roasted wheat.' *(3)*

RIO SALADA. – 'The Spaniards of Rio Salada in South America – who come down from the interior and are employed in transporting goods overland – live wholly on vegetable food. They are very robust and strong, and bear prodigious burdens on their backs, such as require three or four men to place upon them, in knapsacks made of green hides, travelling with a speed which few men can equal without any encumbrance.' *(1)*

BRAZIL, RIO DE JANEIRO, LAGUAYRA. – 'The Brazil slaves are a very strong and robust class of men, and of temperate habits. Their food consists of rice, fruits, and bread of coarse flour and the farrenia root. They endure great hardships, and carry enormous burdens on their heads a distance of a mile without resting. It is a common thing to see them in droves or companies, moving on at a brisk trot, stimulated by the sound of a bell in the hands of the leader, each man bearing upon his head a bag of coffee weighing a hundred and eighty pounds, apparently as if it were a light burden. . . They are seldom known to have a fever or any other sickness . . . The Congo slaves of Rio Janeiro subsist on vegetable food, and are among the finest-looking men in the world. They are six feet high, every way well proportioned, and remarkably athletic. . . The labourers of Laguayra eat no flesh, and are an uncommonly healthy and hardy race. A single man will take a barrel of beef or pork on his shoulders and walk with it from the landing to the custom-house, which is situated on the top of a hill, the ascent of which is too steep for carriages. Their soldiers likewise subsist on vegetable food, and are remarkably fine-looking men.' *(2)*

Similar facts are related of the Peruvians, Tobaso Indians, Kroomen, natives of the New Hebrides, Sandwich Islands, coast clans of the Wamrima, Affghans, Japanese, etc. etc. *(1)*

CYPRUS. – 'It was extraordinary to see the result of a life-long diet of beans and barley bread in the persons of the monks of Trooditissa, who very seldom indulge in flesh. The actual head of the monastery is a handsome man of seventy, perfectly erect in figure, as though fresh from military drill, and as strong as most men at fifty. The younger priests were all good-looking, active, healthy men, who thought nothing of a morning's walk over the fatiguing rocky paths to Troodos and back – twelve miles – to be refreshed on their return by an afternoon's work in their gardens.' *(2)*

'Under the mouldering walls in the recesses of sacred courts, the Moslem cultivates his onion, sugar cane, and fig. . . . . . These dwellers in the plain are good for

more than growing pomegranates and smoking in the shade. Brave, sober, faithful, they have the virtues of a camp. Free of the sword and saddle from their cradles, they are easily turned into good cavalry. No English officer, I am told by experts, would desire a better company before him when he moved into line.' *(3)*

'The people in Cyprus fast more than a third of the year rigorously, only eating bread and vegetables, no milk or oil even. ... A house is considered extravagant where cooking is done more than once in about eight days. Meat and fish are looked upon as rare luxuries. The people look healthy and well, and seem to find enough subsistence in the fruit and herbs that this island produces so plentifully.' *(4)*

ARABIA. – 'Few people surpass the Arabs for longevity, agility, and power of endurance. Yet they subsist on dates and milk, and for months the Bedouin Arabs consume nothing else. The Soumanlies, who inhabit the country in the neighbourhood of Cape Guardafui and Berberah, when on the war path, in which they pass half their lives, live entirely on milk." *(1)*

BOLIVIA. – 'The troopers of this country are fed on maize corn, cocoa, and water. Their strength is surprising and well known. They will perform marches of eighteen, twenty, and twenty-five leagues a day, encumbered with their baggage and without distress.' *(2)*

CANARY ISLANDS. – 'Mr. L. Jewett, of Portland, Maine, says that one of his schooners came into Portland laden with barilla from the Canary Islands ; and that he stood by while the cargo was being discharged, and saw four stout American labourers attempt, in vain, to lift one of the masses of barilla which the captain and mate both solemnly affirmed was brought from the storehouse to the vessel by a single man – a native labourer where they freighted; and he subsisted entirely on coarse vegetable food and fruit' *(3)*

ITALY. – 'The peasants here are a splendid hardy set, living almost entirely upon cakes and porridge of chestnut flour, a little wheat bread, and, at this season, on bread made of the *gran turco* (Indian corn). The country wine is not very plentiful in these parts, and during the last two years the poverty has been too great to admit any drink but water for many families.' *(4)*

CEYLON. – 'The ordinary diet of the people consists of rice seasoned with salt, the chief condiment of the East,

(p. 26)

and a few vegetables, flavoured with lemon juice and pepper, from which they will make at any time a hearty meal ... It is considered anything but a reproach to be sparing in diet' *(1)*

JAPAN. – 'The Japanese not only abstain from animal food, but even from milk and its productions. One of the laws which they most religiously observe is, not to kill, nor to eat anything that is killed. Their chief food consists of rice, pulse, fruits, roots, and herbs, but mostly rice, which they have in great plenty and perfection ; and dress in so many different ways, and give to it such variety of tastes, flavour, and colour, that a stranger would hardly know what he was eating.' *(2)*

'Hot rice cakes are the standard food of the Japanese, and are kept ready at all the inns, to be presented to the traveller the moment he arrives, with tea, and occasionally sacki or rice-beer. The Japanese are represented as robust, well made, and active, remarkably healthy, long-lived and intelligent.' *(3)* Some writers, as in the following extract, observe that the Japanese eat fish. This discrepancy is probably owing to difference of religion, of caste, or perhaps of locality.

'Fish and rice are the staple articles of Japanese diet. The soil is fertile, and apparently vegetables grow well here. Sweet potatoes, ordinary potatoes, turnips, carrots, squashes or pumpkins, egg-plants, and peas are grown, but do not enter largely into the people's diet Beans are an important article, and from these is manufactured *tofee* - literally bean-cheese, an article largely used by the poorer classes. Radishes are also grown, and some varieties are very large and not unlike beets. . . . The young bamboo is also eaten, and a variety of mushrooms is used in making sauces and relishes. . . . Cakes and unleavened bread of various kinds are made from rice flour. ... Of fruits, oranges, peaches, pears, apricots, plums, persimmons, raspberries, mulberries, and currants are indigenous here . . . apples and strawberries have been introduced.... The moisture keeps the vegetation constantly green and beautiful.' *(1)*

SIERRA LEONE. – 'The natives, who live in a climate said to be the worst on earth, are very temperate; they subsist entirely on small quantities of boiled rice, with occasional supplies of fruit, and drink only water; in consequence they are strong and healthy, and live as long as men in the most propitious climates." *(2)*

GREECE. – 'The Greek boatmen are seen in great numbers about the harbours, seeking employment They are exceedingly abstemious ; their food always consists of a small quantity of black bread, made of unbolted rye or wheat-meal, generally rye ; and a bunch of grapes or raisins, or some figs. They are, nevertheless, astonishingly athletic and powerful; and the most nimble, active, graceful, cheerful, and even merry people in the world. At all hours they are singing; blithesome, jovial, and full of hilarity. The labourers in the ship-yards live in the same abstemious and simple manner, and are equally vigorous and active. They breakfast and dine on a small quantity of their coarse bread, and figs, grapes, or raisins. Their supper, if they take any, is still lighter, though they more frequently take no supper, and eat nothing from dinner to breakfast.' *(3)*

MALTA. – 'The Maltese peasant at his best is a model of thrift. Whether he rents a few acres and hires a few hands to assist him in cultivating it, or whether he is himself a hireling, his condition is about the same. He and his family are astir before daybreak, and have not only attended mass, but have also got through two or three hours of hard work in the cool of the morning, before they think about breaking their fast Then another spell of work; and then an afternoon siesta, followed by another turn in the fields and another frugal meal. The system of farming is old-fashioned and oriental, everything being done by handwork, but the soil generally yields each year three crops. The people manage to be strong and hardy on their scanty fare of black bread and coarse macaroni, eked out by such garden stuff as they cannot profitably dispose of in the market, and only washed down on Sundays and saints' days by a draught of the common Sicilian wine, for which they pay two pence a pint. The children who are too young to do rougher work pick the weeds, and these are saved for the goat that supplies them with milk.' *(1)*

TURKEY. – I observed, on a late journey to Constantinople, that the boatmen or rowers of the caïques, who are perhaps the best rowers in the world, drink nothing but water; and they drink that profusely during the hot months of the summer. The boatmen and water-carriers of Constantinople are decidedly, in my opinion, the finest men in Europe, as regards their physical development, and they are all water-drinkers; they may take a little sherbet at times. Their diet is chiefly bread; now and then a cucumber, with cherries, figs, dates, mulberries, or other fruits which are abundant there; now and then a little fish.' *(2)*

'From the day of his irruption into Europe the Turk has always proved himself to be endowed with singularly strong vitality and energy. As a member of a warlike race, he is without equal in Europe in health and hardiness. He can live and fight when soldiers of any other nationality would starve. His excellent physique, his simple habits, his abstinence from intoxicating liquors, and his normal vegetarian diet, enable him to support the greatest hardships, and to exist on the scantiest and simplest food.' *(1)*

'Low stature is the exception in the Ottoman army. These men of herculean form are endowed with fabulous sobriety ; they drink no intoxicating drinks, and seldom touch meat.' *(2)*

'Some of the men among the Turkish excavators were remarkably adroit in throwing up the sand, which they would cast up even as high as twelve feet Their food was of the simplest kind; coarse bread and a little salt fish or olives, black raisins and some fruit occasionally, accompanied by copious draughts of the best water they could obtain, constituted their breakfast and dinner. To their supper, as being the most sumptuous meal, some delicacy, such as thistle-broth, boiled thistle-stalks, snail-soup, dandelion, and other wild vegetables, were often added. With this frugal diet their strength was unusually great, as the fatigues which they endured, in spite of the unhealthy climate, and the great weights which they carried in their arms or on their backs, sufficiently proved. The Turkish porters in Smyrna often carry from four hundred to six hundred pounds weight on their backs, and a merchant one day pointed out to me one of his men who, he assured me, had carried an enormous bale of merchandise weighing eight hundred pounds up an incline into an upper warehouse.' *(1)*

'In Smyrna, where there are no carts or wheel-carriages, the carrying business falls upon the shoulders of the porters, who are seen in great numbers about the wharves and docks and in the streets near the water-side, where they are employed in lading and unlading vessels. They are stout, robust men, of great muscular strength, and carry at one load, upon a pad fitted to their backs, from four hundred to eight hundred pounds. Mr. Langdon, an American merchant residing there, pointed me to one of them in his service, and told me that a short time before, he carried at one load, from the warehouse to the wharf, about twenty-live rods, a box of sugar weighing four hundred pounds, and two sacks of coffee weighing each two hundred pounds, and that, after walking a few rods with a quick step, he stopped and requested that another sack of coffee might be added to his load ; but Mr. Langdon, apprehending danger from so great an exertion, refused his request.' *(2)*

CHINA. – 'The perfection of the art of cooking is nowhere more observable than in the monasteries of the Buddhists. They have but the simplest elements of food to deal with. No meat, no fish, no poultry are allowed at their tables. No eggs, no lard, no butter, no milk must be introduced into their confectionery. Vegetables alone are permitted, and yet by means of these a dinner of surprising variety is served, and if the guest judged only by appearances he would suppose that the worthy abbot had forgotten the rigid rules of his monastic establishment, and was about to break his vow by partaking of most heretical viands.' *(3)*

PALESTINE. – 'The Damascene artisan's or handicraftsman's diet consists of fruit, vegetables, rice, oil, and bread. . . . The diet of both Christian and Moslem is strictly vegetarian, . . . their food is of the most primitive kind, . . . barley or pea bread, with fruit and vegetables.' *(1)*

'The Fellahin, or modern Canaanites, live on simple food; they rarely touch meat, but live on unleavened bread dipped in oil,– reminding one of the poor widow of Sarepta,– or rice, olives, *dibs* (grape treacle), scum (clarified butter), with gourds, melons, marrows, and cucumbers, or, in times of scarcity, the kobberzah or mallow, cooked in some milk or oil. To this frugal diet is due probably the whiteness of their teeth, the strength of their constitutions, and the rapidity with which their wounds heal.' *(2)*

ALGIERS. – 'It was a good beginning to have a stately, barefooted Arab to shoulder our baggage from the port, and wonderful to see the load he carried unassisted. As he winds his way through the narrow and steep slippery streets it is well to see how nobly our Arab bears his load, how beautifully balanced is his lithe figure, and with what grace and ease he walks along. It is generally admitted, we believe, that "a vegetable diet will not produce heroes," and there is certainly a prejudice in England about the value of beef for navvies and others who put muscular power into their work. It is an interesting fact to note, and one which we think speaks volumes for the climate of Algeria, that this gentleman lives almost entirely on fruit, rice, and Indian corn.' *(3)*

AFRICAN COAST. – 'The causeway at Suakin, on the African coast, is the great highway to the interior, and at this season it is daily threaded by long strings of stately camels, with stalwart Hadendoa drivers. You cannot wish to see stouter or better-made men than these fellows, whose glossy skins and well-filled forms show that their diet of dura or sorghum and milk agrees well with them. These two elements compose the food of the whole country side. Milk is in plenty; and of a forenoon in the outskirts of the town one is always meeting a donkey laden with skins of it The dura, which is brought down from the more fertile inland, is not ground in the mill, but by rubbing-stones.' *(1)*

POLAND. – 'Our Polish Upper-Silesians are a very frugal people. A mason who goes to work in the town, distant five to eight English miles or more, must rise in the morning by three o'clock if he will be punctual. His diet for the whole day is the bread which he takes from home in his pocket ... So with the field labourer. As a soldier he is very enduring, and the Polish regiments can always make long marches. The main articles of diet of our Polish peasantry are bread and potatoes.' *(2)*

RUSSIA. – 'Eggs, black bread, milk, and tea – these formed my ordinary articles of food during all my wanderings in Northern Russia. Occasionally potatoes could be had, and afforded the possibility of varying the bill of fare. The favourite materials employed in the Dative cookery are sour cabbage, cucumbers, and kvass – a kind of very small beer made from black bread.' *(3)*

'The people of Russia generally subsist on coarse black rye-bread and garlics . . . . I have often hired men to labour for me in Russia, which they would do from sixteen to eighteen hours for eight cents a day. . . . They would come on board in the morning with a piece of their black bread weighing about a pound, and a bunch of garlics as big as one's fist This was all their nourishment for the day of sixteen or eighteen hours' labour. They were astonishingly powerful and active, and endured severe and protracted labour far beyond any of my men. Some of these men were eighty and even ninety years old, and yet these old men would do more work than any of the middle-aged men belonging to my ship. In handling and stowing away iron, and in stowing away hemp with the jack-screw, they exhibited most astonishing power. They were full of agility, vivacity, and even hilarity, singing as they laboured.' *(1)*

'The Russian peasant is satisfied with the plainest food. . . . The diet consists of pickled cucumbers, cabbages, mushrooms, with a piece of black bread. . . . Unless in the largest towns, butcher's meat would appear to be very little used. Even in such places as Toula and Zaraisk a butcher's shop is never seen. . . . Vegetables and milk compose a great part of the diet in the districts we have now reached.' *(2)*

Here were about 600 irregulars (Russian cavalry), besides militia and regulars, all, especially the irregulars, fine-looking men. The extraordinary thing was that the resources of the country did not seem in any way overtasked to support them; there was no scarcity of anything. As an officer who had served in the French army observed, there was not enough in the place in the way of meat to satisfy two companies of English soldiers, yet here were 3,000 to 4,000 men, many of them of the upper classes. With a little millet boiled into a pudding or "pasta," some goat's milk, cheese, and onions, and a goblet of *"vin du pays,"* even the chiefs are quite contented, while their retainers make good cheer over cake of Indian corn flour, some curds, a piece of dried fish, or a strip of tough beef among half-a-dozen. The Russian soldier is happy with his lump of black bread and glass of whisky or tumbler of weak tea, with, in the evening, perhaps, a basin of weak soup, something like the "black broth" of the Spartans.' *(1)*

NORWAY. – 'The general food of the Norwegians is rye-bread, milk, and cheese. As a particular luxury, peasants eat sharke, which are thin slices of salt hung-meat, dried in the wind, but this indulgence in animal food is very rare indeed. A common treat on high days and holy days consists of a thick hasty-pudding or porridge of oatmeal or ryemeal, seasoned by two or three pickled herrings or salted mackerel All the travellers I have consulted agree in representing the people as thriving on this fare, and in no part of the world are there more instances of extreme longevity than in Norway.'

'Notwithstanding the poor fare of the inhabitants, they are remarkably robust and healthy. Though in many parts of Norway animal food is quite unknown, they are generally tall and good-looking, with a manly openness of manner and countenance, which increased the farther north I proceeded. From this hardy way of living, and being daily accustomed to climb the mountains, they may be said to be in a constant state of training, and their activity is so great that they keep up with ease by the side of your carriage at full speed for the distance often or twelve miles.' *(2)*

SPAIN. – 'With respect to the Moorish porters in Spain, I have witnessed the exceedingly large loads they are in the habit of carrying, and have been struck with astonishment at their muscular powers. Others of the labouring class, particularly those who are in the habit of working on board of ships, and called "stevedores," are also very powerful men. I have seen two of these men stow off a full cargo of wine in casks, after it was hoisted on board and lowered into the hold, with ease. They brought their food on board with them; .t consisted of coarse, brown wheat bread and grapes.' *(1)*

'Those who have penetrated into Spain have probably witnessed to what a distance a Spanish attendant will accompany on foot a traveller's mule or carriage, doing forty or fifty miles a day on his fare of only raw onions and bread.' *(2)*

FRANCE. – 'The way of living in a French peasant's house is this: In the morning the men eat soup, that soup which Cobden praised as the source of French prosperity. It is cheap enough to make. For twelve people two handfuls of dry beans or peas, a few potatoes, a few ounces of fried bacon to give it a taste, a good deal of hot water. The twelve basins are then filled with thin slices of brown bread, and the soup is poured on it Boiled rice, with a little milk, is sometimes taken instead of soup. If the soup is insufficient, the peasant finishes his meal with a piece of dry bread . . . The meal at noon is composed invariably of potatoes, followed by a second dish, which is either a pancake made with a great deal of flour and water and few eggs, or a salad, or clotted milk. No wine or meat is allowed except during the great labours of haymaking and harvest. At these times a little wine is given round with the water drunk at dinner, and a little piece of salted pork.' *(1)*

It is stated in a work published by Bertillon in 1874 that the vine gatherers of the department of Nièvre, of Burgundy, etc, only eat meat once a year, the agricultural labourers of the Maine department eat it twice a year, the weavers of Sarthe on *fête* days only, and the Auvergnese about six times a year. The Breton labourers never eat it, and even rich people in this province take it only on fête days.

SWITZERLAND. – 'The fare of the Swiss workmen is very frugal. They rarely taste flesh, their food being principally bread, cheese, potatoes, vegetables, and fruit; though in the towns the consumption of meat is somewhat greater. The middle classes fare pretty much as the working classes, all consuming large quantities of milk, and drinking coffee mixed with chicory and milk twice a day.

A report upon the alimentation of agricultural labourers in Europe, taken by the order of the English Government, and cited in the 'Anthropological Review' for 1872, gives the following table of dietaries in use among the working populations of various countries:

BELGIUM. – Coffee, brown bread, vegetables, salted bacon. A great number live on potatoes, bread, and chicory plant.

POMERANIA. – Meat (flesh) three times a week.

PRUSSIA (Rhenish). – Milk, soup, dry peas, potatoes, meat on fête days.

SAXONY. – Bread, butter, cheese, soup, vegetables, coffee, meat on fête days.

BAVARIA. – Soup made of flour and butter, milk, cabbage, potatoes.

ITALY. – Macaroni, bread, fruit, vegetables, wine.

LOW COUNTRIES. – Black bread, butter, vegetables, fish, coffee.

RUSSIA. – Rye-bread, cabbage, mushroom soup, buck-wheat baked with milk, oil.

SPAIN. – Bread, vegetables, chick peas; meat is a luxury.

SWEDEN. – Potatoes, rye, oats, barley, abundance of milk, salted herrings, beer; never any meat

SWITZERLAND. – Cheese, milk, coffee, vegetables, soups, wine, rarely any meat They work about thirteen hours a day.

SCOTLAND. – Oatmeal bread, potatoes, milk, butter, coffee, tea, bacon, rarely other meat

IRELAND. – Oatmeal, potatoes, milk, a little lard. A little whisky is also taken.

ENGLAND. – Beef, pork, bacon, potatoes, vegetables, cheese, tea, beer, cider. *(1)*

We see, then, by these examples, that even in our own quarter of the globe, the peasantry and the agriculturists are almost wholly vegetarians in practice, if not by profession and principle. In fact, it is only in England that we find animal food forming part of the regular alimentation of the lower classes. It must not, however, be thought that, even in England, the common use of a mixed diet is equally prevalent in all counties. Mr. Brindley, canal engineer in this country, informs us that 'in the various works in which he has been engaged – where the workmen, being paid by the piece, exerted themselves to earn as much as possible – men from the north of Lancashire and Yorkshire, who adhered to their customary diet of oat-cake and hasty-pudding, with water for their drink, sustained more labour and made larger wages than those who lived on bacon, cheese, and beer – the general diet of labourers in the south.' *(1)* We are, however, aware that the superiority of the English navvies over their French comrades is frequently cited as evidence of the sustaining value of the beef and beer diet of the former, a more meagre fare being, it is said, in use among the Frenchmen. But, supposing the statement to be in all respects correct, it does not appear to involve any anomaly in natural law, for its explanation lies in the fact that the Saxon workmen belong to a sturdier, a hardier, and a more staying race than the Celts whose most remarkable exploits are generally accomplished under the influence of passing emotion or enthusiasm. The Frenchman excels, not in physical power or muscular development, but in agility and Man; he is concentrated in performance but quickly exhausted; the Englishman, on the contrary, is dogged, tenacious, and enduring. It is much more likely that the English navvy owes his superior working power to the hereditary gifts of his race than to an accidental use of certain comestibles to which, by the bye, his forefathers were strangers. But it is not contended that stimulating substances, such as alcohol and flesh, may not temporarily give rise to a display of excessive energy, and that under their influence a man may not perform feats which would be well-nigh impossible to him in an unexcited condition – as a person pursued by a bull will leap a five-barred gate which, in cooler moments, he would be forced to climb. And if any man affirm that beef and beer enable him to accomplish labour other-wise beyond his strength, the fact may be attributed, not to increase of muscular force, or development of stamina, but to quickened nervous action, or stimulation.

Formerly, indeed, the diet of the country labouring classes was almost wholly innocent of flesh-meats and strong drinks, and it must be borne in mind that it is to this sober and temperate ancestry that the working powers of the present generation are owing. The use of flesh as daily food dates from hardly more than a quarter of a century among the peasantry of most rural districts, and already they are beginning to degenerate. The children will have neither the health nor the constitution of their fathers, nor their immunity from suffering. In Mr. Smiles's 'Life of George Moore,' we read that in old times even the well-to-do country classes were strangers to the taste of flesh, and that 'stalwart sons and comely maidens were brought up on porridge, oatcakes, bannocks, potato-pot and milk.'

A native of Maine (France) informs me that in his grandfather's time the peasants of that department enjoyed far longer life and more robust health than the present generation who have exchanged the simple sustenance of former years for a dietary consisting largely of stimulating drinks and animal food. Examples of this kind are not far to seek and might be indefinitely multiplied, whether with regard to races, communities, or families.

If from national generalities we pass to the consideration of individual experience of the Pythagorean system, we are met by such an enormous mass of evidence as would require volumes to chronicle it. Let a few instances, chosen from thousands, suffice; the limits of this little treatise preclude more numerous citations.

'The celebrated Lord Heathfield, who defended the fortress of Gibraltar with consummate skill and persevering fortitude, was well known for his hardy habits of military discipline. He neither ate animal food nor drank wine; his constant diet being bread and vegetables, and his drink, water.'

'My health,' says Mr. Jackson, a distinguished surgeon in the British army, 'has been tried in all ways and climates; and by the aid of temperance and hard work, I have worn out two campaigns and probably could wear out another. I eat no animal food, drink no wine, malt liquors, nor spirits of any kind. I wear no flannel, and regard neither wind nor rain, heat nor cold.'

'Professor Lawrence knew a lady who, having adopted a vegetarian mode of life, was remarkable for her activity and strength. She made nothing of walking ten miles, and could with ease walk twenty. She had two children, and nursed them for about twelve months each, during which time she took only vegetables and fruit, with distilled water as drink. Both children were fine and healthy.'

'Another lady (the wife of one of the founders of the Vegetarian Society in England) abstained from flesh and all intoxicants for thirty years, and during that time, gave birth to fifteen children, fourteen of whom she nursed herself, and yet remained young and active.' *(1)*

The celebrated reformer of the eighteenth century, John Wesley, wrote to the Bishop of London in 1747, that, following the advice of Dr. Cheyne, he had given up

(p. 41)

the use of flesh-meat and wine, and that from that time, 'thanks to God,' he had been delivered from all physical ills.

In the month of October, 1878, a Jewish rabbi named Hirsch Guttman, died at Gross-Strehlitz at the advanced age of 108 years. He had been a vegetarian for half a century. Rabbi Guttman was presented to the Emperor of Germany, who, after a long conversation with the old man, respectfully received his blessing. *(1)*

Since, then, we find that the exterior structure of mankind, their internal organism, their natural instincts and the habits of the greatest ancient races, as well as the modern experience of so many nations and communities in every part of the globe, all plead in favour of an alimentation derived immediately from the fruits and seeds of the earth as the most nutritious and proper to humanity, it would indeed be anomalous if the results of chemical analysis were to show themselves less favourable to the same conclusion. Let us see, then, what chemistry has to say on the subject.

FOOTNOTES

(18:2) Rollin's Ancient History, vol i.
(21:1) Smith's Fruits and Farinacea.
(21:2) Lane's Egypt.
(21:3) Catherwood.
(21:4) Buckle's History of Civilisation.
(21:5) Elphinstone's History of India.
(22:1) Lyon's Residence in Mexico. 1838.
(22:2) Taylor's Selections from Humboldt's Works on Mexico, 1824.
(22:3) Sir Francis Head, also Dr. Lyon Playfair and Darwin.
(23:1) Smith's Fruits and Farinacea, 1850.
(23:2) Graham's Lectures.
(24:1) Sir John Sinclair, Graham, Pope, Cook, Burton, and Buckingham.
(24:2) Sir Samuel Baker's Cyprus in 1879.
(24:3) Hepworth Dixon on the Island of Cyprus.
(24:4) Standard, Article on Cyprus.
(25:1) Lieutenant C. R. Low in the *Food Journal.* 1873.
(25:2) Panama Star and Herald.
(25:3) Smith's Fruits and Farinacea.
(25:4) Private letter from Lucca.
(26:1) Pridham's Ceylon, 1849.
(26:2) Mod. Univer. Hist., also Smith's Fruit and Farinacea.
(26:3) Smith.
(27:1) New York World, 1877.
(27:2) Monthly Magazine, 1815.
(27:3) Judge Woodruff of Connecticut.
(28:1) One and All, also Dietetic Reformer, 1880.
(28:2) Sir William Fairbairn's Report on Sanitary Conditions.
(29:1) Standard, 1877.
(29:2) Daily News, 1877.
(30:1) *Discoveries at Ephesus.* by F. T. Wood, F.S.A., 1877.
(30:2) Judge Woodruff.
(30:3) *Pictures of the Chinese,* by the Rev. R. H. Cobbold. M. A.
(31:1) Official Report of Acting Consul.
(31:2) Tent-work in Palestine, by C. R. Conder, R.E., 1878.
(31:3) Artists and Arabs, by Henry Blackburne, 1868.
(32:1) By the Red Sea, Professor Robertson Smith.
(32:2) E. Wellshaenser.
(32:3) Dr. Mackenzie Wallace's Russia.
(33:1) Capt. C. S. Howland, of New Bedford, Mass.
(33:2) Bremner's Excursions in the Interior of Russia.

(34:1) War Correspondent of the Daily News, 1878.
(34:2) Dr. Capell Brooke and Mr. Twining.
(35:1) Capt. C. F. Chase.
(35:2) Smith's Fruits and Farinacea.
(36:1) Hamerton's Round my House, 1875.
(36:2) Leisure Hour, 1873.

(37:1) Add to the above, that many religious communities in all eliminates systematically abstain from flesh-meats. For instance. S. Benedict's rule prohibits the flesh of quadrupeds to all except the feeble and sick. The rule of S. Francis of Paula is severely vegetarian, forbidding; even eggs and milk. The Trappist monks, the religious of S. Dominic's order (friar preachers), and of S. Basil's order, are all vegetarian; and among the orders of women, the rule of life of the Poor Clares is similar. Apart from religion, there exist also numerous bodies professing Pythagoreanism. To instance one or two of these only, the Vegetarian Society of England, established in 1846, numbers over 3,000 members; the Food Reform Society of London has a large following, and there are several vegetarian restaurants in the metropolis. Vegetarian societies exist also in Paris, Switzerland, Germany, America, etc., etc.

(38:1) Smith's Fruits and Farinacea.
(40:1) Smith.
(41:1) Dietetic Reformer

5. CHEMISTRY

All the various alimentary substances divide themselves naturally into two groups, organic and inorganic, the organic group being subdivided into substances containing nitrogen, and those which do not contain it These last again divide themselves into fatty bodies, composed of carbon and hydrogen, combined with a very small proportion only of oxygen; and into carbohydrates, which are also constituted by carbon united to hydrogen and oxygen, but in which the two latter elements always exist in the same proportion as they do in water ($H^{10} O^5$). Such are the polymeric bodies, gum, cellulose, dextrine, starch, etc. Glucose, which forms the solid and crystallisable part of honey, and which exists in the greater number of dried fruits, on the surface of which it forms efflorescences, is represented by the formula, $C^6H^{10}O^5 + H^2O$ – that is to say, it is the ultimate product of the transformation of cellulose, and, more particularly, of starch. One molecule of dextrine, in absorbing two molecules of water, gives two molecules of glucose. Levulose, which is found in a great number of fruits, and galactose, are isometric with glucose; the formula of saccharose or cane-sugar and of its isometric body, lactose, or sugar of milk, is represented by two molecules of glucose, less one of water.

There exist, however, some few substances which do not find a place in this classification, such as alcohol, pectine, and the vegetable acids. Alcohol occupies an intermediate rank between the fatty bodies and the carbo-hydrates, while the other substances mentioned are still more highly oxydised than the carbo-hydrates.

Some chemists class together all the non-nitrogenised substances, i.e. fatty bodies and hydrates of carbon, under the general name of hydro-carbons; but although this classification may, from certain points of view, have the merit of convenience, it is wanting in clearness and precision. All the carbo-hydrates are largely present in vegetable and fruit produce, but, if we except sugar of milk (lactine), and muscle-sugar (inosite), none of the group belong to healthy animal tissue. On the contrary, the true hydro-carbons, consisting of a fatty acid in combination with a radical, occur equally in animal and in vegetable matter. Of these fatty bodies, that known as 'stearine' is peculiar to animal substances, while both kingdoms are rich in 'palmatine' and 'oleine,' the latter, as fluid fat, being, however, chiefly present in vegetable products. *(1)*

It was formerly taught by Liebig that the destiny of nitrogenised principles in the animal economy was quite distinct from that of the non-nitrogenised principles. According to this theory the first contributed to the growth and nutrition of the elements of the animal economy, and to the production of muscular and nervous force while the last served only as fabricants of heat, and were accordingly named 'respiratory' elements of food.

It is now known, that in making this classification Liebig erred, and that neither is the action of nitrogenised principles exclusively limited to nutrition, nor that of fatty matters to the production of heat In fact the latter, although particularly heat producers, take their part also in the work of nutrition, and, far from being so restricted in their operation as was supposed, it is now proved that the fatty bodies constitute the true source of physical force, and that they may be fairly styled the generators of motor power; while to the nitrogenised principles appears to be reserved the function of giving birth to those elements which make part of the composition of the animal organism itself Now, certain recent and numerous experiments made, not on the lower animals, but on man himself, and having therefore considerable value, demonstrate that the production of force is not due to the oxydation of the nitrogenised element of the living tissues of the organism, as was formerly believed by those who thought with Liebig, bur, on the contrary, to the oxydation of hydro-carbonated substances. Therefore the production of mechanical force, like that of heat, is the result of the oxydation of the elements of carbon and hydrogen; the energy set free by chemical action manifesting itself under the form of mechanical force. *(1)*

The fatty bodies, properly so called – stearine, palmatine, and oleine – fulfil, then, equally the part of force-producers and that which Liebig assigned exclusively to them, of producers of caloric. Now, the capacity to produce heat depends on the quantity of carbon and hydrogen not already oxydised, which exists in any given substance, and this condition is, in a special degree, realised in the composition of fatty bodies. It is from this point of view that it is necessary to distinguish between the hydro-carbons – fatty bodies – and the carbo- hydrates – starchy and sugary bodies – because these last contain a proportion of oxygen sufficient in itself to oxydise all the hydrogen contained in them, leaving the carbon only unoxydised; while in the fatty bodies, not only the carbon, but the larger part of the hydrogen also, remain unoxydised.

As regards the utilisation of the carbo-hydrates, it is under the ultimate form of sugar that they all finally enter the economy. It may be said that while the saliva and the pancreatic juice play the first part in the conversion of starch into sugar, it is the liver that takes the initiative in the assimilation of the sugar, and this action apparently gives birth to the amyloid, colloid, or non-diffusible substance known as glycogen, a substance which itself in its rum is converted into hydro-carbonated or fatty matter. *(1)*

It is, then, under the final form of fatty matter that starchy and sugary substances act as heat producers. This transformation is probably attained by a giving off of carbonic acid and oxygen, which process would leave of the composition of a carbo-hydrate the chemical formula only of a fatty body: $- C^{12}H^{10}O^9 - CO^2{}_2O - C^{11}H^{10}O$.

It must be borne in mind that, as producers of force, sugar, and its anterior forms, such as dextrine, gum, and starch, possess only the value of the quantity of oxydisable and non-oxydised substance which they contain.

Coming to the consideration of nitrogenised principles, we find that they exist equally in animal and vegetable articles of food, and that, whichever may be their origin in nature, they are absolutely identical Vegetable albumen is obtained most abundantly from the cereals, and in smaller quantities from nuts and leguminous plants ; vegetable fibrine is obtained by washing the flour of the cereals, in which it forms part of the substance known as crude gluten, and. is separable from the pure gluten by treatment with boiling alcohol It exists also in grape juice, and in the majority of leguminous plants. Vegetable caseine is found in great quantity in all kinds of beans, peas, and other seeds, and is often spoken of as legumine. It is present also with albumen in almonds and other oily grains.

There remain yet two organic nitrogenised substances, the source of which is exclusively animal, and which form a separate group, readily distinguishable from that just described, by the fact that they do not give proteine by the action of heat and an alkali, as do the albuminous, fibrinous, and caseinous substances. These principles, gelatine and chondrine, are derived from bone and fibrous animal tissues, cartilage, ligamentous and tendonous material, and by them is constituted the jelly of flesh-meat soups. *(1)* Their nutritive value has been greatly disputed, and was the subject of a special inquiry instituted by the Academy of Sciences of Paris, forty years ago. The conclusions arrived at by the commission appointed to examine the question, tended to demonstrate that the food-value of gelatinous compounds, if not absolutely nil, was at least extremely doubtful Bischoff and Voit, however, more lately (1874) have given an opinion that these substances may cover proteid waste, and to some slight extent form a substitute, by admixture, for other plastic matter.

The special action of the proteinous nitrogenised principles is, as we have already seen, to furnish elements, first for the development, and, secondly, for the renewal, of the tissues of the animal organism. These proteinous principles serve also in the. production of the secretions of the economy; and as the amount of the secretions bears proportional relation to the vital activity, it is easy to understand how necessary to the integrity of the animal functions is the ingestion of such principles.

To complete our sketch of the nature and destiny of the elements which enter into alimentary compounds, it remains to say a few words on their inorganic constituents. These, under the form of mineral salts and mater, are indispensable to the nutrition of living beings. Of these substances the principal are the combinations of lime, magnesia, potash, sod's iron, the chlorides, and phosphoric, carbonic, and sulphuric acid, lime and he phosphates being, perhaps, the most essential The part taken in the animal organism by water and saline matters appears to consist chiefly in contributing to establish the conditions necessary to the production of the chemical action, by the aid of which proteid and other substances are assimilated, and in forming the liquid part of he bodily humours. (The serum or water of the blood, a slightly albuminous liquid, amounts in the human body to about three litres in quantity.) Salts do not appear to be themselves capable of acting as force producers, but they form an essential part in the composition of all the humours and secretions, and exist in combination with the organic principles in every animal tissue. The various salts necessary to complete alimentation are present alike in vegetables and in flesh. In the vegetable kingdom the largest proportion of phosphates, chlorides, and potash is met with in the cereals, and it is worthy of remark that these salts, as well as the nitrogenised elements, are present principally in the tegument or exterior part of the grain, and, consequently, ordinary white bread contains but a comparatively small proportion of them. In order to obtain the full value of Jour, it should be eaten unbolted–that is to say, the meal should be used entire, and not deprived, by dressing, of its tegumentary parts.

Water furnishes us with chloride of sodium, carbonate of lime, and silex; iron is largely present in peas, haricots, and lentils; the herbs and leguminous vegetables are rich in phosphates of lime.

By means of the following table, the composition of the various alimentary substances most in use, of both vegetable and animal origin, and their comparative nutritive values, may be readily perceived and understood. The analyses given are those of Fresenius, Letheby, Pavy, Church, Wolff, Knop, and Payen: – IN 100 PARTS

	Nitrogenous Matter	Hydro-carbonate Matter	Saline Matter	Water
Lean beef	19.3	3.6	5.1	72.0
Fat beef	14.8	29.8	4.4	51.0
Lean mutton	18.3	4.9	4.8	72.0
Fat mutton	12.4	31.1	3.5	53.0
Veal	16.5	15.8	4.7	63.0
Fat pork	9.8	48.9	2.3	39.0
Dried ham	8.8	73.3	2.9	15.0
Tripe	13.2	16.4	2.4	68.0
White fish	18.1	2.9	1.0	78.0
Red fish (salmon)	16.1	5.5	1.4	77.0
Oysters	14010	1515	2695	80385
Mussels	11.72	2.42	2.73	75.74
White of egg	20.4	...	1.6	78.0
Yolk of egg	16.0	30.7	1.3	52.0
Cow's milk (Lactine 5.2)	4.1	3.9	0.8	86.0

Cream (Lactine 2.8)	2.7	26.7	1.8	66.0
Butter	...	83.0	2.0	15.0
Gruyère cheese	31.5	24.0	3.0	40.0
Roquefort cheese	26.52	30.14	5.07	34.55
Dutch cheese	29.13	27.54		36.10
Chester cheese	25.99	26.34	4.16	35.92
Parmesan cheese	44.08	15.95	5.72	27.56
Cheddar cheese	28.4	31.1	4.5	36.0

IN 100 PARTS

	Carbo-Hydrates	Nitrogenous Matter	Hydro-Carbonate Matter	Saline Matter	Water
Beans	55.86	30.8	2.0	3.65	8.40
White haricots	557	25.5	2.8	3.2	9.9
Dried peas	587	23.8	2.1	2.1	8.3

Lentils	56.0	25.2	2.6	2.3	11.5
Potatoes	21.9	2.50	0.11	1.26	74.0
Black truffles	16.0	8775	560	207	72.0
Mushrooms	3.0	4680	396	458	91010
Carrots	14.5	1.3	0.2	1.0	83.0
Sea-kale	2.8	2.4	...	(?) 3.0	93.3
Turnips	7.2	1.1	...	0.6	91.0
Cabbage	5.8	2.0	0.5	0.7	91.0
Garden beet	13.5	.4	...	(?) 1.0	82.2
Tomato	6.0	1.4	...	(?) .8	898
Sweet potato	26.25	1.50	.30	2.60	67.50
Water-cress	3.2	1.7	...	(?) .7	93.1
Arrow-root	82.0	...	...	...	18.0
Dry southern wheat	67112	22.75	2.61	3.02	...

Dry common wheat	77.05	15.25	1.95	2.75	...
Oat-meal	63.8	12.6	5.6	3.0	15.0
Barley-meal.	74.3	6.3	2.4	2.0	15.0
Rye-meal	73.2	8.0	2.0	1.8	15.0
Dry maize	71.55	12.50	8.80	1.25	...
Dry rice	89.65	7.55	0.80	0.90	...
Buckwheat	6490	13.10	3.0	2 50	13.0
Quinoa-meal	56.80	20.0	5.0	(?) 1.0	15.0
Dhoora-meal	74.0	90	2.6	2.3	...
Dried figs	65.9	6.1	0.9	2.3	17.5
Dates	65.3	6.6	0.2	1.6	20.8
Bananas	(?) 19.0	4820	632	791	73900
Walnuts (peeled)	8.9	12.5	3.6	(?) 1.7	44.5

Filberts	11.1	8.4	28.5	(?)1.5	48.0
Ground-nuts (peeled)	11.7	24.5	50.0	(?)1.8	7.5
Cocoa-nut	8.1	5.5	35.9	(?)1.0	46.6
Fresh chestnuts (peeled)	42.7	3.0	2.5	(?)1.8	49.2
Locust bean	67.9	7.1	1.1	(?)2.9	14.6
Cocoa-nibs Chocolate	11.10	21.20	50.0	3.0	12.0

Fresh fruits of the drupaceous, baccate, and pomaceous classes – plums, peaches, olives, cherries, grapes, currants, cranberries, gooseberries, oranges, citrons, apples, pears, etc., etc. – contain a very large proportion of carbo-hydrates, vegetable acids, salts, and water.

We have it, then, clearly demonstrated by the foregoing analysis, that not only do vegetable substances contain all the elements necessary to nutrition and to the production of force and heat, but that they contain proportionately even more of these elements than are found in animal substances. For instance, peas, beans, lentils, and haricots contain from 23 to 30 per cent of proteid matter, 55 to 58 of starch, and about 3 of saline matter, while animal food contains from 8 to 19 of proteid matter and no carbo-hydrates at all. Fatty matter, is however, present to a larger extent in flesh meats than in ordinary vegetable and grain produce, but the use of seed and nut oils abundantly compensates for this deficiency. We have it shown also, that not only are the nutritive and dynamic values of vegetable foods, taken in their totality, greater than those of animal foods, taken in their totality, but that the former contain, besides, a whole class of principles which do not exist in the composition of the latter. These are the carbo-hydrates, the relative place of which in human alimentation we shall presently see. And if to vegetable produce proper, are added certain other aliments, which, though of animal origin, may, without inconsistency, be introduced into a Pythagorean regimen – such as milk, eggs, cream, butter, and cheese – we have at our disposition the entire range of the very substances which, of all aliments known to man, are richest in nitrogen and hydro-carbons. I say 'without inconsistency,' because:

(1) All animals of the order to which man himself belongs, are nourished during their infancy by milk, the derivatives of which cannot therefore be regarded as improper to their or his nutrition;

(2), because all these substances, especially cheese and curds, habitually formed part of the diet of the ancient phytivorous peoples;

(3), because morality is in nowise outraged by their use;

(4), because, as we shall see further on, their use is not excluded by economical considerations.

As regards the proportional quantity of each principle which should enter into the daily alimentation of man, it varies according to sex, circumstances, and personal habit. On the average, in a state of repose or with moderate exercise, the proportion should be –

	Oz.
Nitrogenous matter	4.215
Hydro-carbons	397
Carbo-hydrates	18.090
Salts	0.714

During active exercise and prolonged work, as with manual labourers, soldiers engaged in war, etc, the proportion should be –

	Oz.
Nitrogenous matter	5.41
Hydro-carbons	2.41
Carbo-hydrates	17.92
Salts	0.68

Let it be noticed that these dietaries, which are quoted from Dr. Playfair, contain a large proportion of carbohydrates – substances which, as we have seen, do not exist in the food of carnivorous animals, for no animal tissues in the healthy state contain them; the few traces of incite in muscular fibre not being worth mention. They are found principally in fresh fruits. The carbo-hydrates are absolutely necessary to proper human alimentation; they take the place which would otherwise be occupied by fatty matter, and their use prevents fatigue of the digestive organs. Moreover, fruit acids possess certain proper qualities which appear to exercise on the economy a special influence – purifying, cooling, refreshing, corrective, regulatory – such as no other substances are able to supply.

FOOTNOTES
(42:1) Pavy.
(43:1) The following observations occur in the works of Dr. Flint Professor of Physiology at the hospital of Bellevue. New York (*Experiments and Reflections upon Animal Heat*, 1879). He remarks that the calorific value of any article of food may be expressed by a definite number of unities of caloric. Of these unities a certain proportion is converted into force, which divides itself into muscular force and respiratory and circulatory force. Professor Foster (*Text-book of Physiology*, 1877) has calculated that a fifth or sixth pan of the total value of any aliment is employed under the form of muscular force, the other four-fifths or five-sixths which remain being converted into heat. Now, according to Joule, the unity of caloric (i.e. the quantity necessary to raise one degree Fahrenheit a pound weight of water) equals the force necessary to raise one foot in height 772 pounds ('*Mechanical Equivalent of Heat*.' *Philosophical Transactions*, 1850). Therefore, muscular force results from the transformation of the heat produced in the organism after the appropriation of a quantity of caloric sufficient for the maintenance of the constant animal temperature. The oxydation of the elements of carbon and hydrogen is a much more important factor of calorification than that of nitrogen, for it is certain that the calorific value of the oxydation of the first two, and the quantity of heat thus produced, are much more considerable than in the case of the oxydation of nitrogen. It is probable, according to Dr. Flint (who does not, however, altogether accept the conclusions of his authors), that a production of caloric is always going on in the living organism, even in the absence of any alimentation. The heat thus produced would be. according to his experiments, the result of the oxydation of the hydrogen forming miter with the oxygen inspired into the lungs. Of this oxygen, eighty-six parts in a hundred combine with carbon to form carbonic acid. The value of the caloric thus obtained must be added to the calorics obtained by the ingestion of food in order to arrive at a just calculation of the quantity of heat and dynamic force which the organism has at its disposal, under such or such conditions.
(45:1) Pavy.
(46:1) Fruit and vegetable jelly is formed by pectine and pectic add, and is therefore of a totally different nature from that yielded by bone stock.

6. STIMULATING EFFECTS OF FLESH FOOD

But, if it is indisputably demonstrable that the alimentation afforded by a vegetable diet is more efficacious, more varied, richer in nutritive and dynamic principles and more fitted to the requirements of 'man than flesh-meats, the superiority of which, from all these points of view, has been so long maintained, it is also possible to adduce evidence of facts tending to prove that the use of animal viands produces an effect analogous to that of alcohol; that they stimulate and excite the nervous system ; that they rapidly waste its elements, as also those of all the organism; and that they thus indirectly diminish vital resistance and the term of natural life. And though it might be deemed exaggeration to say that the use of flesh-meats induces premature death, it is certainly true that it hastens the arrival of old age, and the manifestation of diseases and diatheses, as much by its directly baneful effects on the system, as by the habits it engenders, such as alcoholism, unchastity, and excesses of all kinds. Referring to the immediate effects on the nervous system of the ingestion of flesh-meats, Dr. Pavy says: –

'Animal food exerts a greater stimulating effect upon the system than vegetable fare. Accounts are related of the stimulant properties of animal food having sufficed, in those accustomed only to a vegetable diet, to produce a state resembling intoxication. Dr. Dundas Thompson *(1)* quotes a narrative of the effects of a repast of meat on some native Indians, whose customary fare, as is usual amongst the tribe, had consisted only of vegetable food. They dined most luxuriously, stuffing themselves as if they were never to eat again. After an hour or two, to his greet surprise and amusement, the expression of their countenances, their jabbering and gesticulations, showed clearly that the feast had produced the same effect as any intoxicating spirit or drug. The second treat was attended with the same result.'

Dr. Druitt, also, *(1)* describing the properties of a liquid essence of beef prepared according to his instructions, speaks of it as exerting a rapid and remarkable stimulating power over the brain, and introduces it to notice as an auxiliary to, and partial substitute for, brandy, in all cases of exhaustion or weakness, attended with cerebral depression or despondency. Correspondingly stimulating properties have been claimed as the effect of other similar compounds. I myself once knew a young lady of nervous temperament, who but very seldom ventured to partake of more than a single plate of animal viands at the same meal, for fear of becoming surexcited. One day, being very hungry, she transgressed her rule and ate two mutton chops, and, as I happened to be seated beside her, I witnessed the result of this excess, which soon avenged itself in the shape of a fit of actual intoxication. It is certain that the conduct even of beasts may be modified by the character of their food. In the '*Lancet*' *(2)* Liebig maintains that the ingestion of flesh produces in the carnivorous races the ferocious and quarrelsome disposition which distinguishes them from the herb-eaters. A bear, kept at the Anatomical Museum of Giessen, showed a quiet gentle nature so long as he was fed exclusively on bread, but a few days' feeding on meat made him vicious and even quite dangerous. It is well known that swine grow irascible by having flesh-food given them, and under such conditions will attack men; and that dogs kept for the purpose of protecting houses and other premises are often fed upon flesh expressly to render them ferocious and combative, and dangerous therefore to burglars. Blood-hounds, fox-hounds, and indeed all animals used for pursuit or attack are similarly fed, while the domestic skye-terrier or pug, if he is to be gentle and 'sweet' both physically and morally, must be nourished on a biscuit and bread-and-milk diet Examples of this kind are of the commonest experience; rather than multiply them it is preferable to occupy ourselves with their explanation.

Dulong asserts that the quantity of oxygen 'lost' during respiration – that is, the quantity not replaced by carbonic acid – constitutes in the herbivora about a tenth part of the volume of the quantity utilised and replaced by carbonic acid; and in the carnivora he has found that the quantity of oxygen thus 'lost' varies from a fifth to half the whole quantity. And Drs. Fife and Spalding have demonstrated by experiment that in the same individual, a mixed diet necessitates a greater consumption of oxygen than a vegetable diet, the respiratory movements being more frequent in the former than in the latter case. These facts prove, Dr. Craigie thinks *(1)* that flesh-food gives rise to more violent and laborious pulmonary action than alimentation by vegetable diet.

Again, in his '*Animal Chemistry*,' Liebig calls attention to the restlessness and incessant movements of carnivorous animals, lions, tigers, hyenas, etc., in the menageries, and observes that men who are habitually kreophagist manifest similar irritability and want of repose.

This condition of high pressure in the vital processes ought, doubtless, to be referred to the particular manner in which the absorption of the elements of flesh-food takes place, these elements, as we have seen, comprising no carbo-hydrates. In fact, the work of digestion and assimilation appears to be much more rapid in the case of animal alimentation, and consequently, as has been already said, a proportional vital exhaustion and break-up of organic tissue ensues. Now, the digestion of flesh takes place principally in the stomach, while that of the principles dominating in vegetable products occurs to a great extent in the intestine. Therefore, digestion and assimilation are more complex and less rapid processes in the latter case, and the function of absorption is, so to speak, more extended and generalised than it is when dealing with animal food, which taxes the stomach almost exclusively. It is chiefly to this rapid and precocious absorption of the nitrogenised principles predominant in flesh, as well as to the lack of the moderating and regulatory effect of the carbohydrates, that I am disposed to attribute that exciting influence of animal alimentation which has been already mentioned, an excitation, which, like that produced by the ingestion of alcohol, passes quickly away and impels to a renewal of the sensation so soon as the stomach is emptied of its consents. Let us be careful to distinguish between this condition of functional excitement and true invigoration. How many persons deceive themselves in this respect, and think they are strengthened and reinforced when they are only stimulated! Who has not witnessed, particularly during the convalescence following typhoid fever, the phenomenon known as *febris carnis*, an ephemeral fever which shows itself after the first flesh-meat meal administered to a patient recovering from serious illness, and which is sometimes the occasion of a relapse! This phenomenon is, probably, due at least in great pan to the rapid absorption of the proteinous principles of animal food, though this may not be the exclusive cause of the disturbance; but in the present state of our chemical knowledge it is not possible to affirm that these principles themselves – globuline, myosine, syntonine, etc – may be taken to contain some subtle evanescent element capable of explaining more completely the stimulating and intoxicating effects to which, attention has been called. However this may be, it is certainly to the absence of this sensation of stimulation habitual to flesh-eaters, that must be attributed the 'sinking,' the languor, the weakness even, which in the majority of cases is experienced by them during the first few days following a change to vegetable diet Symptoms, precisely similar, are witnessed in persons addicted to alcoholism, when deprived of their spirituous drinks; and in both cases, the sensations described disappear more or less rapidly, according to circumstances and individuals, under persistent treatment But many persons, misled by this passing feebleness, and mistaking its nature, fancy that they are losing strength, and after three or four days' abstinence from flesh, return to their former habits. In order to avoid this factitious weakness, it is strongly urged on kreophagists, as well as on alcohol-drinkers who desire to change their mode of life, to wean themselves from it gradually and by progressive steps, until little by little they arrive at the adoption of an absolutely reformed regimen.

FOOTNOTES

(52:1) Experimental Researches on the Food of Animals.
   (53:1) Transactions of the Obstetrical Society, 1861.
   (53:2) Vol. i. 1869.
   (54:1) Elements of the Practice of Physic, vol. ii.

7. ALCOHOLISM

Allusion has already been made to the deplorable *indirect* effects of flesh-eating. Of these alcoholism is one of the commonest. An American reformer, who for more than forty years has occupied himself in lecturing on the subject of dipsomania, and who, since the commencement of his career, has carefully noted the causes of this disease in an immense number of persons of all classes in the many various countries and climates he has visited, avers without reserve, that the use of flesh-foods, by the excitation which it exercises on the nervous system, prepares the way for habits of intemperance in drink, and that, other things being equal, the more flesh is consumed the greater is the temptation to make use of strong pungent drinks, and the more serious is the danger of confirmed alcoholism. Many experienced physicians have made similar observations, and wisely act on them in their treatment of dipsomaniacs. *(1)*

Dr. Austin Flint, of Harvard Medical College, is of opinion that the use of flesh-meat ought always to be forbidden in all cases of acute or chronic gastritis, because the stimulating properties of flesh are invariably ill-supported by a diseased and enfeebled stomach. Now we know that chronic gastritis always, sooner or later, accompanies alcoholism, and that one of its symptoms is excessive thirst, which in aggravated cases becomes well-nigh continuous. There is in this state of things a regular circle of cause and effect Animal viands keep up the gastritis by over-stimulation and taxation of the affected organ; the gastritis excites thirst; thirst perpetuates drunkenness. And, since we know that the dominant principles of flesh are precisely those the digestion of which is effected in the stomach, it will easily be understood how injurious to a diseased or ailing organ, already degenerated or enfeebled, must be the prolonged and exclusive labour imposed upon it by a highly nitrogenised regimen.

Dr. Jackson, senior physician of an asylum for inebriates at Dansville (United States), observes that he always found it impossible to benefit his patients permanently so long as they were permitted animal food, the use of which be regards as an absolute barrier to a radical cure. It is evident, he thinks, that flesh contains some extra-alimentary principles, which excite the nervous system to such a degree that it ends by exhausting and degenerating it so as to deprive it of all vital power. This condition of exhaustion, he adds, gives rise to a paroxysm of craving for abnormal stimulus, and the desire for alcohol is thus renewed and sustained. Every patient who places himself under Dr. Jackson's care is therefore required to conform to the rules of the asylum, and to abstain entirely from animal viands of all kinds, as well as from tea, coffee, and tobacco. Under these conditions, says Dr. Jackson, a man cannot help becoming sober and regenerate, it being impossible for him to live six months exclusively on unbolted meal bread, vegetables, and ripe fruit, such as apples, pears, apricots, peaches, etc, without entirely ridding himself of the fever of alcoholism. Such a regimen completely renovates the system and destroys the appetite for strong drinks; evidence of which facts, continues Dr. Jackson, may be witnessed at any time in the establishment of which he has charge, the treatment there pursued excluding entirely the use of drugs, and relying solely on the regulation of diet and the use of baths.

Next, in regard to other allied excesses, it is certainly not difficult to understand that the stimulation and irritation produced in the nervous centres by the constant ingestion of highly nitrogenised and exciting meats, influences the genital functions in a powerful degree, and sets up a condition of pressing insatiability. Not to dwell on the details of this part of our subject, let it suffice to observe, in passing, that the deepest, truest, and most general causes of prostitution in all great cities must be looked for in the luxurious and intemperate habits of eating and drinking prevalent among the rich and well-to-do. The chief element of this luxury is the use of flesh and alcohol, which mistaken notions of hygiene and therapeutics tend to press more and more upon all classes of men and women. Abolish kreophagy and its companion vice, alcoholism, and more, a thousand-fold, will be done to abolish prostitution than can be achieved by any other means soever as long as these two evil influences flourish. The young man of the present day, accustomed from childhood to frequent and copious meals of flesh, and from early youth to the use of all manner of fermented beverages and liqueurs, carries about with him and fosters an increasingly disordered appetite, which not infrequently assumes the character of true disease, destroying all capacity for the duties and the higher pleasures of intellectual and refined life.

FOOTNOTES

(57:1) Vegetarianism the Radical Cure for Intemperance, H. B. Fowler. New York.

8. SLAUGHTER-HOUSES

And now, as belonging to the same class of evils indirectly due to flesh-eating, we shall speak of the very serious inconvenience and impediments to civilisation caused by the existence of Slaughter-Houses. These establishments, even when submitted to regular surveillance, are apt to become sources of sickness and epidemic complaints, particularly when they are placed in the neighbourhood of large towns and during the hot season. In the 'Times' of July ii, 1874, a correspondent – Mr. Samuel A. Barnett – thus describes the dangers and horrors of these disgusting institutions: –

'It is impossible for any but those who live and work near here to understand all the suffering which the Whitechapel and Aldgate slaughter-houses entail. To reach these houses the cattle have to be driven along a street crowded with trams, omnibuses, and general traffic. The drivers are almost of necessity cruel, as they hasten the brutes through such a thoroughfare; the animals, excited by shouts and blows, frequently make frantic rushes, and endanger the lives of the foot-passengers. From these slaughter-houses, too, the blood flows across the pavement, and there arises a close smell which seems to thicken the air and make breathing a pain.... We know that life here is not vigorous; the air has no refreshing power; and we are well able to understand why so many resort to drink. Dr. Liddle, our medical officer, has spoken and written strongly on the harm done to the health of our neighbourhood by means of these houses. The medical officers of the Health Association have, I think, agreed unanimously on the injurious effect of the trade. Those who crowd our courts, the passers through our streets, the little children who see the cruelty, the cattle who suffer, all want a voice to tell their needs. It is out of my power to do more than ask your help. By your means the House of Lords may learn the meaning of an Act which establishes slaughter-houses in the City. I trust we may not have a law directly injurious to health passed by a Government whose motto is *sanitas sanitatum.*'

Mr. Brooke Lambert, late Vicar of St. Mark's, Whitechapel, followed up the preceding letter with these corroborative statements: –

'If any one wishes to know whether the nuisance be real, let him turn out of the Whitechapel Road at the entrance to the London and North-

Western goods station, and pass down the streets leading thence to Man-sell Street. He will then know what the smell of blood is. And yet he will probably often boldly encounter the smell of blood in preference to the worse sights he will risk in Whitechapel Road. The carts laden with fresh skins, the pails full of blood and brains, are sights to which a long experience does not harden one. 'Another correspondent, with a dash of keener insight than the others seem to possess, writes: –

'I am quite convinced that all these disgusting sights and sounds, from which no care can secure our poor children, *are inseparable from the thing itself*'

With this last expression of opinion all logically minded persons must concur. In whatever locality the slaughter-house may be erected, there the noxious odours, the revolting cruelty, the degrading sights, the unwholesome atmosphere, the pathetic cries, the perpetual bloodshed, and all the attendant accumulation of sickening horrors will inevitably abound. Nor have men of culture and education any right to raise an outcry against the conduct of a trade while daily sustaining themselves on its produce. Picture the writer of any one of the foregoing protests, after having despatched his letter to the 'Times' office, sitting down complacently to enjoy his slice of sirloin or of saddle of mutton!

9. SOCIAL CONSIDERATIONS

And here we come face to face with a momentous question, supremely interesting from the point of view of human rights.

Is it morally lawful for cultivated and refined persons to impose upon a whole class of the population a disgusting, brutalising, and unwholesome occupation, which is scientifically and experimentally demonstrable to be not merely entirely needless, but absolutely inimical to the best interests of the human race?

Butchers are the Pariahs of the western world; the very name itself of their trade has become a synonym for barbarity, and is used as a term of reproach in speaking of persons notorious for brutality, coarseness, or love of bloodshed. The common exclamation, 'What a butcher is So-and-so!' in reference to such men, betrays the horror and reprobation with which are instinctively regarded the followers of a trade created and patronised chiefly by the 'refined' classes!

In the report of a 'diseased meat' case given in the 'Leeds Mercury' of March 6, 1880, the ensuing passage occurs: –

'Mr. J. Ellis, President of the Leeds Butchers' Association, stated that there was no disease about the lungs of the animal at all. Blood had probably been forced into them by some person jumping on the animal's body after it had been felled.

'Mr. Bruce: Is it a common practice *when a beast is dying* for a person to jump upon it to force the blood out of it? Witness: Yes.'

In the course of the celebrated Tichborne case a certain metropolitan butcher was called to testify to the claimant's identity. This man averred that *employés* in slaughter-houses habitually make use of clogs to avoid soaking their feet in the pools of blood which continually inundate the pavements of these places. Really, when one thinks of these unfortunate and brutalised men, thus condemned by modern 'civilisation' – Heaven save the mark! – to pass their days in the midst of spectacles and practices so foul and loathsome, taking part daily in wholesale massacres, and living only to take away life, it is impossible not to conclude that such men are deprived of all chance of becoming themselves civilised, and are consequently disinherited of their human rights, and defrauded of their human dignity. And not only the slaughterers themselves, but all those who are directly or indirectly associated with this abominable traffic – cattle-drivers and dealers, meat-salesmen, their apprentices and clerks – all these live in. familiar, if not exclusive, contact with practices and sights of the vilest and most hideous kind; all these are condemned to the degradation or suppression of the most characteristic features of Humanity.

With people in general the very look and touch of raw flesh excite a disgust which only a special education can overcome. So that in the butcher and cook persons are condemned to work which their employers deem - altogether repulsive. It is absurd to suppose that if kreophagy were really natural to mankind, the sentiments in regard to butchers and their trade, to which allusion has been made, would find such spontaneous and universal expression among us. The true carnivora and omnivora have no horror of dead bodies, the sight of blood, the smell of raw flesh, inspires them with no manner of disgust If all of us, men and women alike, were compelled to dispense with the offices of a paid slaughterer and to immolate our victims with our own hands, the *penchant* for flesh would not long survive in polite society. It would be indeed hard to find a man or woman of the upper or middle classes who would willingly consent to undertake the butcher's duties, and go to the cattle-yard armed with pole axe or knife to fell an ox or to slit the throat of a sheep or lamb, or even of a rabbit, for the morrow's repast On the other hand, there is no one, however delicately bred or refined, who would not readily take a basket and gather apples in an orchard or peaches in a garden, or who, if need should arise, would object to make a cake or an omelette.

It would, alas! require many long pages to cite the innumerable cruelties and sufferings which the gluttony and luxury of flesh-eating man impose on the innocent herb-feeders – sufferings which, whatever may be said to the contrary, are *absolutely inevitable and* inseparable from modem European habits of diet Sufferings by sea and land, in transit from different ports, by rail and by road, sufferings in the live-stock markets, in the pens of the slaughter-houses while waiting their turn for death, sufferings by thirst, starvation, sickness, overcrowding, cold, heat, mutilation, blows, terror, apprehension, exhaustion, neglect, to say nothing of the wanton barbarity to which they are too often subjected, such, under the present hateful and unnatural system, is the woful lot of the patient, gentle, laborious creatures who should be ploughing our fields, and yielding us, not their flesh and blood, but milk and wool and the fruits of their willing toil.

See these details, taken from the report of the Veterinary Department of the Privy Council for the year 1879. The reporter draws attention to the enormous losses of American cattle caused by the miseries of the Transatlantic passage, and the same complaint is reiterated in the report for last year.

In 1879, 157 cargoes of Canadian cattle were shipped for Bristol, Glasgow, Liverpool, and London, in which total there were 25, 185 oxen, 73, 913 sheep, and 3, 663 pigs. Out of this number *154* oxen, 1, 623 sheep, and 249 pigs were thrown into the sea during the passage; 21 oxen, 226 sheep, and 3 pigs were landed dead; and 4 oxen and 61 sheep were so wounded and suffering on arriving that they had to be slaughtered on the spot.

In the same year there were shipped from the United States for the ports of Bristol, Cardiff, Glasgow, Grimsby, Hartlepool, Hull, Leith, Liverpool, London, Newcastle-on-Tyne, South Shields, and Southampton 535 cargoes of animals, of which 76, 117 were oxen, 119, 350 sheep, and 15, 180 pigs. Out of this number 3, 140 oxen, 5, 915 sheep, and 2, 943 pigs were cast into the sea during the transit; 221 oxen, 386 sheep, and 392 pigs arrived dead at the place of landing, and 93 oxen, 167 sheep, and 130 pigs were so mutilated that they had to be sacrificed on the spot In *résumé*, 14,024 animals were thrown into the sea, 1,240 were landed dead, and 455 were slaughtered on the quay to save them from dying of their wounds and sufferings.

10. SUFFERINGS OF THE CATTLE

A clergyman writes *(1)* that being on board a vessel bound from Madagascar with 160 cattle on deck and the same number in the hold, a storm came on, and the deck was cleared by throwing the animals into the sea. Sharks crowded round, tearing the bullocks limb from limb. The poor creatures charged the vessel in their efforts to escape, and clambered as far as they were able up the ship's side, only to fall back again bellowing and panting into the waves. The sea was red with blood, and the sight awful to witness. The hatches were battened down, and all the cattle in the hold were suffocated. Everyone on board was ill from the stench caused by the corpses. 'A friend to whom I told this,' says the writer, 'informed me that once coming from Hamburg on a ship with 220 sheep on board, 200 were thrown into the sea, and the remaining twenty were landed more dead than alive.'

A recent paragraph in the '*Daily Telegraph*' says: – 'If certain rumours respecting the intolerable sufferings to which homed cattle are subjected during their transport from America to this country be founded on fact, it is high time that the Board of Trade turn its serious attention to obtaining official protection for the unfortunate creatures doomed to the horrors of a long sea voyage with the shambles as its goal, in order that English tables may be plentifully supplied with fresh beef.

Under favourable weather conditions a bullock passes its time on board ship in a chronic condition of fear and misery; but when the winds blow and the vessel rolls heavily, the agonies it suffers are such that their mere contemplation might melt a heart of stone. That wilful torture should be permitted to aggravate the already unbearable torments to which a severe gale condemns these wretched beasts appears incredible; yet we have been assured that expedients of such dire cruelty that we forbear from shocking the public by describing them, are mercilessly put in practice in order to *compel oxen, maddened by sheer physical pain, to leap overboard* when the movement of the vessel is so violent as to preclude the possibility of their being dealt with by the crew. It is a significant fact that, within the last few days, a vessel which left the shores of America with a cargo of 594 live bullocks arrived in the port of London with only 45 of its homed passengers, the other 549 having perished in consequence of heavy weather!'

And, of the land transit of cattle, Mr. Street, agent of the American Humane Association, writes: –

'The official reports of the different railway companies prove that thousands of animals arrive at stations dead, and thousands more in a crippled and tortured condition, with broken limbs and horns. We have seen ten or twelve drays from morning to noon hauling away the dead and maimed victims at a single station. The hogs that have broken backs or limbs are dragged by their ears and tails to be "loaded" upon trucks and hauled to the slaughter-houses. The cattle in the cars, which cannot rise to their feet, yet are still alive, are pulled out and left to lie upon the platform until they are sold to men who buy dead and injured animals. I have travelled more than 18,000 miles, and have visited 1,340 local stations where cattle are collected and shipped. I saw at the Kansas station large fine-looking oxen which the owner expected to sell for exportation, that had been confined in small pens for three days and nights continuously exposed to the hot sun, and the cold, *without food or water.* The man in charge said that he was instructed by the owner to give them no food or water, as be expected, when they reached St Louis, *to get one hundred pounds or more of water into each before they were sold and weighed.* A large number of the shippers told us that they never allowed their cattle to have food or water for at least twenty-four hours before putting them In the can, because cattle kept hungry and thirsty did not incline to lie down. In the torment of hunger and thirst, however, the larger beasts often turn restive, and the smaller fall or lie down and are trampled to death by their fellows.'

Mr. Edward Byron Nicholson, M.A., principal Librarian and Superintendent of the London Institution, has very lately published an 'Essay on Ethics,' in which the following passage occurs: –

'There is no need to *see* whether the slaughter of a pig is swift and painless or not But I have watched the slaughter of oxen and sheep. The animals were kept waiting some time in a slaughter-house round which (at least in the case of the sheep) were hung carcases and Kins of their fellows, so that they could hardly have helped seeing what lay in store for them. The oxen had to be hauled about with ropes fastened to their heads to put them into the fit position. Each animal was then felled with a poleaxe, which did not take away its feeling, and, *while it lay groaning, a piece of wood was worked round in its brain.* I think the sheep's throats were cut without their being felled. Other sheep were standing outside in the yard, seeing, and hearing through the wide-open door the bleats of their dying mates. These are not at all picked cases: I saw them in the slaughter- house of one of the largest butchers in a good-sized town within thirty miles of London.'

Lastly, to terminate evidence which might be almost indefinitely multiplied, let the reader study the following extract from the letter of a 'Journeyman Butcher' which appeared in the 'Staffordshire Daily Sentinel' of June 17, 1879: –

'The first lessons a butcher's apprentice generally receives from the journeyman is how to torture the animals which are to be slaughtered; and they are frequently allowed to use the axe before they are well able to lift it, to the indescribable agony of the poor beast. Again, when a slaughterman is in a hurry to get away he is not particular about skinning the animal before it is dead. This I have seen occur daily, where there has been a large amount of work to be done. I have seen slaughtermen make bets which would first have five or ten sheep (as the case might be) killed, skinned, and hung up. You may depend they were not particular about them being dead before they commenced to skin. I have seen cows knocked down and their heads severed from the body almost immediately, while the muscles and the flesh have been quivering. When an animal is being driven into the slaughter-house it is generally very restive, in consequence of the blood, etc., it sees about. Then it has to undergo a large amount of kicking on the legs, tail-twisting, and stands a chance of getting a horn knocked off *I have seen their eyes burst and their tails sawn before they could be got inside*. There is another species of cruelty of a different kind. Animals are frequently brought from a distance and put in the «clemming" house for perhaps *a couple of days without water of food*. . . . I could mention other cruelties that are frequently practised, but I think this enough to show the public what is daily occurring in our slaughter-houses. The society with a long name' (Royal Society for the Prevention of Cruelty to Animals) 'and the police are almost powerless, as a deal of slaughtering is done very early in the morning, and with closed doors, particularly in the winter.'

The editor of the *'Sentinel'* adds by way of commentary on this naive and rugged epistle: –

'Habit blunts the sensibilities of men who are not naturally cruel; and, besides, there are many people who never realise the fact that "brute beasts" can be made to suffer at all. People who would look with horror at the torture of a man, complacently behold the sufferings of his poor relations. We are afraid that the pleasures of the table would be greatly impaired if the guests knew the whole history of the manner in which the steaming joint or the daintily-served chicken even, had been prepared for their use. 'Tis enough to make vegetarians of us all even to think of it.'

No wonder that with the facts we have recounted before his eyes, Dr. Richardson, of hygienic fame, at a recent public congress, expressed his 'sincere hope that before the close of the century, not only would slaughter-houses be abolished, but that all use of flesh as food would be absolutely abandoned.' *(1)*

And again, in a paper read at a meeting of the Sanitary Congress, the same well-known lecturer, describing his Utopian country, *'Salut-land,'* or *'Hygeia,'* said: –

'In the midst of the towns the eye is struck with the cultivation of fruit-trees that prevails. The towns of Salut-land might be called, as ancient

Norwich once was called, the towns or cities of orchards. Throughout all the country the land is under cultivation of the most perfect kind for cereal produce and fruit and vegetables. . . . A man, woman, or child who for wanton pleasure should hunt down or torture one of the inferior creatures would be cast out of society, while the idea of having dumb animals killed and hung up in open shops to bleed and be quartered and cooked for human beings to live on, would be treated with disgust.'

And a 'Parish Parson,' in a letter which appeared in a serial publication for February 1881, sums up the butcher and slaughter-house question very fairly and concisely in these words: –

'The moral considerations press us on two sides with irresistible force. The aggregate of animal suffering in the cause of the table is simply appalling, and there is nothing for it but to shut our eyes and ears. The life of an ox from the pasture to the butcher's shop will not bear telling. One night on a cattle-steamer would be enough for most of us. The table. . . . brutalises and degrades a multitude of men whom society employs and shuns ... To the craftsman, the tiller, the market-dealer any intelligence and virtue is possible. One might live in a worse place than Covent Garden, and the booksellers do not seem out of place there, nor children in the way of much moral hurt But the "meat market!" And so all our ideas of life and its dignity and significance suffer, and our relations to the animals keep, and must keep, a depressed level. Of course, if all this is inevitable, it is. If all this suffering and depraving are essential to health and happiness, they must go on. But of this creed believers dwindle and skeptics. multiply. The "good dinner" seems likely to be at last the "scientific frontier" of the question, and when it comes to that it will be the beginning of the end.'

FOOTNOTES

(65:1) Dietetic Reformer, June 1880.
(69:1) Dundee Advertaiser, 1879.

11. DANGERS OF FLESH-EATING

And now let us quit this subject, so briefly glanced at, of the indirect evils of kreophagy, to examine some of those *direct* deplorable effects of the custom, which present themselves under the form of various diseases and cachectic bodily conditions.

These, in the first place, are due to a bad condition of the flesh-tissue consumed. Now flesh may be rendered bad, and dangerous to the eater:

(1) By the existence in it of parasitic disease;

(2) by other diseases having during life affected the animal from which it is taken;

(3) by poisons ingested by the animal during life;

(4) by decomposition of the flesh after death.

Flesh infested by parasites infects the eater of it almost invariably. The *cysticercus cellulosæ* of the pig constitutes perhaps the commonest example of this kind of infection. It appears to be very widespread among Irish swine, for, according to Professor Gamgee, *(1)* from three to five per cent of these animals are found to be infected with this particular malady. The cysticercus of the bullock and calf is smaller than that of the pig, and more difficult to discern. Flesh thus affected cannot be rendered safe food by any process of salting or smoking; and even the temperature of boiling water, although it kills the parasite, is only effective when every particle of the tissue throughout its entire thickness has been submitted to an equal heat In the digestive organs of the man who has the misfortune to eat meat thus infected, the cysticerci develop into the large tape-like intestinal worms known as taenia. The cysticercus of the pig produces the *taenia solium*; that of the ox and the calf the *taenia medio-canellata*.

Yet another form of parasitic disease, known as *trichina spiralis,* exists in butcher's meat, and is more common in pork than in the flesh of other animals. This terrible malady was in 1863 the cause of a disastrous event in Helstadt, Prussia, A hundred and three persons, having at one meal partaken of a dish of sausages made of infected pork, were attacked with trichinosis, and more than twenty of the sufferers died within a month. Trichinosis is not uncommon in countries where pork is largely eaten, especially where it is eaten salted or smoked. To destroy trichinae a temperature of at least 212° (Fah.) is needed, and this heat, of course, must penetrate every atom of the flesh-fibre. The manifestations of the disease are at first similar to those of typhoid fever; subsequently atrocious pains make themselves felt in every muscle of the body; the patient lies moaning constantly and unable to extend the limbs on account of the agony caused by the least movement; and death occurs in the midst of symptoms resembling those of cholera, or of pneumonia or some other inflammatory disorder. No case is known of a radical cure, for, even if the unfortunate sufferer escape death, the parasites encyst themselves, and thus remain indefinitely imprisoned in calcareous envelopes in the muscular tissue.

Besides parasitical diseases, cattle may be affected by acute malignant diseases, such as rinderpest, pleuro-pneumonia, anthrax, and simpler inflammatory disorders. Professor Gamgee's statistics in the report already cited show that a fifth of the total quantity of flesh-meat consumed is derived from animals killed in a state of disease, malignant or chronic.

It has been affirmed that little danger attends the ingestion of the flesh of such diseased beasts, but a remarkable case adduced by Mr. Simon in the report to the Privy Council proves this assertion. to be ill-founded. A heifer on a farm in Aberdeenshire, being somewhat out of health, was slaughtered by a ploughman and a blacksmith. Fart of the animal's flesh was cooked next day for the dinner of the family, consisting of eleven persons. Nine of these partook of the meat, and were all soon seized with such alarming symptoms of poisoning that a medical man was at once called in. Two of the patients died. A few days later both the ploughman and the blacksmith were admitted to the Aberdeen Royal Infirmary, suffering from phlegmonous erysipelas of the arm. The offal of the slaughtered heifer had been cast on a dung-heap, to which two swine had access. They ate freely of it, and both were seized with sickness and died.

A similar case occurred in January 1878, and was the subject of a coroner's inquiry in West Kent On the 31st of that month a bullock belonging to a farmer at Addington was observed lying down, apparently ill, in its stall. The animal's throat was cut immediately, and a butcher named Bell, assisted by another man, dressed the carcase. Some days afterwards Bell complained of pain in his right arm, which was considerably swollen, and Dr. Booth, of Beckenham, pronounced the symptoms to be those of blood poisoning. Bell gradually became worse, and died on February 12. It appeared that at the time of dressing the carcase Bell had two slight scratches, one on the hand, the other on the arm. It was supposed that the bullock had been suffering from cattle disease, and that the abrasions of his skin had allowed some of the animal's vitiated blood to enter his system.

The bailiff who cut the bullock's throat, and in doing so got some of its blood sprinkled over him, was attacked about the same time as Bell with similar symptoms, but in his case medical treatment proved successful The man who had assisted Bell in flaying the carcase was also affected with pain and indisposition. About a week afterwards, a pig which had been in the farmyard was found dead, and it is thought it may have been killed by eating the offal or blood of the dead bullock. Mr. Hill, the owner of the animal, and his bailiff denied that previously to the bullock's death there had been any indication whatever of disease among the cattle on the farm. *(1)*

Sir Robert Christison, M.D., asserts positively that the flesh and secretions (milk included) of animals affected with carbuncular disease analogous to anthrax, are so poisonous that those alike who handle and who partake of them are apt to suffer severely, the disease taking the form either of inflammation of the digestive canal, or of an eruption of one or more large carbuncles. Dr. Livingstone also, in his 'Missionary Travels and Researches in South Africa,' speaks of malignant carbuncle – anthrax – occurring as a result of eating the flesh of diseased animals.

In the spring of 1841, four members of a family, after having partaken of a sheep affected with an ordinary cattle disorder, were attacked with symptoms of severe irritant poisoning, and one of them died in less than three hours. A labourer at Horsham and two of his children died in June 1844 from eating flesh similarly vitiated. During the month of April 1879, a Zurich tribunal was occupied for three days with a case in which a butcher and an innkeeper were charged with the sale of veal from calves suffering with typhus. The meat was consumed by the members of a choral society, six of whom died, while six hundred and forty-three suffered more or less severely.

Or. A. Carpenter, speaking before the Sanitary Congress already mentioned, said that he had heard an agent of the police, Inspector of the Metropolitan Meat Market, assert upon oath, that *eighty per cent*, of the flesh meat sent to the London market is affected with tubercular disease; and he added that to exclude such meat from the trade would leave the public without a meat supply!

Again, ruminants, and still more often rabbits and hares, may during life consume some vegetable or other substance of a poisonous nature, and their flesh may thus be rendered dangerous as food for man. It is worthy of remark that certain animals may themselves eat with impunity herbs or fruits, and yet after death set up symptoms of poisoning of a violent character in the human consumer of their flesh. In the 'Edinburgh Medical and Surgical Journal' (July 1844) it is observed, that 'in America there are certain regions extending for many miles in length and breadth, on the herbage of which, if an animal feeds, its milk and flesh acquire poisonous properties, yet itself enjoying tolerable health.' The flesh of rodents fed upon belladonna, or rhododendron chrysanthemum, which these animals eat without injury to themselves, is undoubtedly dangerous to the life of the consumer.

FOOTNOTES

(71:1) Fifth Report of the Medical Officer to the Privy Council.
(74:1) Daily Telegraph.

12. TREATMENT OF DISEASE

We come next to the disastrous effects produced by the ingestion of flesh-meat in a tainted or partly decomposed condition; effects which are frequently observed and therefore well-known. Their symptomatology is that of gastroenteritis (inflammation of the stomach and intestine), often accompanied by fever and sometimes very severe. *(1)* Death not infrequently terminates these cases. In the brief space of a *fortnight,* occurring in the month of October 1879, the quantity of putrefied butcher's meat seized by the police in the London Central Meat Market amounted to seven and a half tons, besides three tons of bams, bacon, and tongues also declared 'unfit for human food.' 'If this be the state of affairs in one particular market, the quantity of putrid flesh which finds its way into the hands of consumers in places where no such strict supervision is maintained, must,' says the 'Edinburgh Evening News,' 'be something enormous.' Statistics on this subject are common in all the daily papers, and it is not worth while to crowd these pages by reproducing them.

Animal-meat may thus directly engender many painful, loathsome, and fatal disorders. Nor is it less demonstrable that it is also in a less direct manner, the origin of a vast number of maladies and pathological diatheses. Scrofula itself, that fecund source of suffering, deformity, and death, not improbably owes its origin to kreophagite habits. It is curious that the root of the word scrofula is *scrofa* – a sow. To say that a person is scrofulous is then to say that he has the *swine's evil.* We know how common is the use of pork among all classes of our population, and especially among the poor. Bacon, sausages, and lard are components of almost every meal of the lower and middle classes, both in town and country. *(1)*

Of all the ultimate manifestations of the strumous or scrofulous diathesis – of which almost everybody in our part of the world bears traces in some form – *tubercular phthisis* is at once the commonest and the deadliest. Dr. Buchan observes that this malady, so prevalent in England, appears to be due to the excessive use of animal food, and advises that 'when there is a tendency to consumption in the young, it should be counteracted by strictly adhering to a diet of the farinacea and ripe fruits. Animal food and fermented liquors ought to be rigidly prohibited.' This opinion coincides exactly with that of Dr. Lamb, who expresses his own views in almost identical terms. Drs. Bannister (United States) and Pemberton are also partisans of the treatment of scrofula, and all strumous manifestations, by a diet of milk, farinacea, and strict exclusion of all flesh-foods. The following case is recorded by Dr. Knight, of Truro: –

'Two years ago I was applied to by Mrs. A— affected with scrofulous ulceration of the left breast. The ulcer was then the size of a half-dollar, and discharging a considerable quantity of imperfect pus. The axillary glands were much enlarged, and, doubting the practicability of operating with the knife in such cases, I told her the danger of her complaint, and ordered her to subsist upon bread and milk and fruit, to drink water, and keep the body of as uniform a temperature as possible. I ordered the sore to be kept clean by ablutions of tepid water. In less than three months the ulcer was healed, and her general health much improved. The axillary glands are still enlarged, though less so than formerly; she still lives simply and enjoys good health, but tells me that if she takes flesh-meat, it produces "twinging" in the old sore.' In the *'Lancet'* for May 14, 1842, is recorded the following case of complete cure of severe strumous ulceration in a child three years of age, by Mr. Rowbotham of Stockport: – 'The little son of Mr. Fielding of that town had been ill eighteen months. He was covered from head to foot with ulcers; his eyes, nose, ears, mouth, and, in fact, his whole head and face, were involved in one complete mass of fetid running sores and ulcers; and the lower part of his body was in a similar condition, so that the thighs seemed almost separating from the body. For more than twelve months the boy had been quite blind; and had never been able to sit down, even on a pillow, but stood, and leaned with his elbow on his nurse, except at times when he was able to kneel on a pillow; he had scarcely been able to lie in bed for the same period. Eight of the most eminent medical men had declared the case hopeless, and some thought that it was not even capable of amelioration. "From certain views which I held on the origin of disease," says Mr. Rowbotham, "I was induced to recommend a diet consisting almost entirely of ripe fruits, and honey, sugar, or treacle. The child commenced this diet on September 13, 1841; he had stewed fruits, mixed with sugar or honey, at all his meals, and was allowed frequently to eat grapes, cherries, plums, apples, pears, and such other fruits as could be obtained. On the 16th, the sores on his back were beginning to heal; on the 23rd he was sensibly improved; on the 30th one half of his face was clear; the lower parts of his body were much better, and he could sit in a chair and lie comfortably in bed He continued daily to improve, till at last his eyes opened, but they were at first very weak, and he could scarcely see anything; his sight however, gradually improved. On January 1, 1842, not a single ulcer remained on his body; the skin became remarkably dear and fair; and the features – which, for twelve months, had been in such a state that it was impossible to do more than guess at the position of the nose and eyes –

were restored to their wonted appearance." *(1)*

Dr. Pavy *(1)* thinks that a regimen rich in carbo-hydrates would be the most suitable in cases of tubercular diathesis, and observes that the want of these substances is probably a main cause of the development of tubercle. Now, we know that the carbo-hydrates are contained solely in the products of the vegetable kingdom, and particularly in fruits. With regard to the action of hydro-carbons (fatty bodies) in scrofula, Dr. Pavy inclines to look on them as absolutely indispensable. Since experience shows the beneficial effects of these substances, systematically employed, in scrofulous and tubercular diathesis, it is only reasonable to infer, says Dr. Pavy, that a measure which proves efficacious in removing an unhealthy condition would also tend to prevent its development Notwithstanding the plain inference of such wise observation, we see daily in our hospitals, and often in private practice, tuberculous patients undergoing a disgusting and unwholesome 'treatment' by *raw meat*, on the pretext that this substance is more easily and rapidly assimilated than any other kind of food. It is true that this is the case; but what is the reason and what the effect of this rapid assimilation?

The reason is that the dissolution of flesh takes place wholly in the stomach, and consequently its digestion is soon accomplished; the effect is the production of that condition of general. excitation peculiar to diffusible stimulants, to which attention has already been called in these pages – an excitation whose ultimate result can only be to precipitate the manifestation of the hectic fever which is the chief characteristic of tuberculous cachexia, and which the physician ought, on the contrary, to combat as determinedly and as long as possible. *(1)* Besides, in such cases, as Dr. Pavy well remarks, a highly nitrogenised alimentation, once assimilated and passed into the organism, becomes even more injurious from another point of view. It gives rise, in fact, as we shall presently see, to the formation of products which require for their elimination a very considerable amount of labour on the part of the kidneys – labour which ought, in cases of inflammatory disease, to be avoided. The carbo-hydrates and the fatty substances, on the contrary, impose no work on these organs; the products of their utilisation, consisting of water and carbonic acid, leave the organism by other channels. The now well-known experiments of Lehmann on himself, and of Messrs. Lawes and Gilbert upon cattle, show that the proportion of urea in the urine is in direct ratio to the quantity of nitrogenised food consumed.

While subsisting on an exclusively animal diet, Lehmann eliminated in twenty-four hours 53.2 grammes (820 grains) of urea; on an exclusively vegetable diet, 22.5 grammes (347 grains) of urea were eliminated; on a mixed diet, 32.5 grammes (501 grains); and, finally, upon a diet composed solely of non-nitrogenous substances – hydro-carbons and starchy matter – only 15.4 grammes (237 grains) of urea were eliminated in the twenty-four hours. These figures are calculated upon an average of twelve observations in each case. Lehmann affirms that five-sixths of the nitrogen contained in ingested aliments pass into the urine under the form of urea. For instance, having absorbed 30.16 grammes of nitrogen a day, 25 grammes of it were excreted in urea during the twenty-four hours. According to these data it follows that ingested nitrogenous matter must undergo in the economy certain metamorphoses of which urea represents the ultimate result That these metamorphoses take place with great rapidity is demonstrated not only by Lehmann's experience, but by analogous experiments conducted by Dr. Parkes upon two soldiers. Lehmann asserts further, that animal food raises the proportion of fibrine contained in the blood, and we know that during inflammatory processes this element exists in it to a large extent, especially in acute rheumatism and pneumonia, ten parts of fibrine per thousand having been found in the blood in cases of the former, and six or nine per thousand in cases of the latter malady – the normal proportion being three per thousand parts. And whenever, in the course of a disorder of another nature, an inflammatory process is set up in any organ, the same phenomenon is observable. *(1)*

It may perhaps be objected that as the residue of a hydro-carbonaceous and carbo-hydraceous alimentation (the ultimate action of the last being identically the same as that of the fatty substances) is eliminated chiefly by the skin, such a dietary might, by increasing the pathological sweats, prove injurious in phthisical cases. Let it be observed in reply that these sweatings are really due to the ingestion, not of hydro-carbons, but of nitrogenised matter, for these last, by the rapidity with which their assimilation is accomplished, and by the stimulating action they set up, kindle and accelerate feverish action, and that the febrile access ceases as soon as the sweats appear, for by their agency Nature relieves herself of the toxic element It is then by the skin that the fever is eliminated, and a sweat not provoked by feverish process cannot be dangerous to the consumptive patient, but might rather, for *rationale* and mode of action, though in a far milder degree, be compared to the Turkish bath, to the beneficial effect of which in cases of tubercular diathesis frequent testimony has been borne.

These facts explain also why the ordinary mixed food is less suitable than a milk and vegetable diet to the treatment of chronic *nephritis*.

In the case of a mixed alimentation the greater portion of the solid matter contained in the urine is composed of the nitrogenised products of the flesh-substances ingested. Now, when any particular organ of the body is ailing, it appears reasonable to diminish as much as possible the amount of work imposed on it, and, adopting this view, we may hope, by the use of a vegetable regimen, avoiding of course all such strongly proteinaceous food as beans, lentils, etc., to succeed in formulating a wise dietary treatment of Bright's disease. Semola, a physician of Naples, proscribes in this malady *all* nitrogenous aliments, and advises an exclusively feculent regimen. *(1)* Besides, and from another point of view, bearing in mind the relation between certain alimentary compounds and the production of urea, we ought also in Bright's disease to guard against the ingestion of nitrogenous and quickly assimilable substances, which, by giving rise to copious and rapid formation of urea, may hasten the manifestation of uraemia.

There is yet another diathesis, the most appropriate and complete treatment of which consists in the prohibition of all flesh-meats. I speak of *gouty* diathesis. One of the effects of animal alimentation is to provoke a condition of acidity of the urine, while the use of vegetable diet renders it alkaline. The ordinary reaction of human urine is acid, and it is customary to call this the normal reaction, because it is that which is met with almost exclusively among populations nourished on a mixed diet But the reaction becomes neutral or alkaline when the use of animal food is abandoned, and with the acidity disappear also the concretions, which, in accumulating, constitute lithiasis. *(1)* The quality of the ingesta has then an enormous influence on the production of gravel; and we know that uric acid, the presence of which in excess constitutes the essential character of uric lithiasis and of gout, results from the imperfect combustion of nitrogenous matters, for these, being incompletely oxydised, form uric acid instead of the urea which would be normally produced. We must then expect to find in persons addicted to the ingestion of large quantities of animal food, an excess of uric acid, and consequently a tendency to gout, calculi, and nephretic colic. In order, therefore, to escape the development of these disorders, so often hereditary, as well as to treat them when already manifested, a vegetable diet is distinctly indicated. *(2)*

Dr. Craigie, in his *'Elements of the Practice of Physic,'* says: – 'A diet consisting of bread and milk or rice and milk, or the flour of farinaceous seeds and milk, is quite adequate to prevent the formation of the gouty diathesis, and to extinguish that diathesis, if already formed Such diet is also adequate to prevent the disease from appearing in its irregular form, and affecting the brain and its membranes, or the heart and lungs. If further arguments were required in proof of the position that milk and grain diet (not in large quantity), or diet of boiled vegetables and milk, while both necessary and adequate to the cure of gout, is perfectly safe, and much less injurious than diet of animal food, they may be found in the facts observed in the physiological relation between the stomach on the one hand and the lungs on the other.'

Dr. Cullen entertains the same opinion; and Dr. Cheyne informs us that the Prince of Condé was cured of obstinate gout by the adoption of a regimen excluding all forms of fish, flesh, and wine.

According to Dr. Cullen, not only gout, but *rheumatism,* should properly be treated by the same method, for he adds that the cure of this latter malady requires in the first place an antiphlogistic regimen, and particularly total abstinence from animal food – a statement which seems reasonable enough when viewed in connection with the facts noted by Lehmann in regard to the increase in the quantity of fibrine in the blood under an animal regimen, for we have seen that this element tends to augment enormously in rheumatism.

Diabetes mellitus is a disease in the treatment of which it has become classic to prescribe an almost exclusively flesh-meat diet, as being the only one which contains no carbo-hydrates. But it must be remembered that, whatever regimen may be adopted, the urine of the diabetic patient will continue to contain sugar – a fact which in itself suffices to prove that the presence of sugar in the urine is but a symptom of a disease having its cause in a morbid condition which probably existed a long time before its manifestation. In what then did this morbid condition consist? Here is a problem which has never yet been satisfactorily solved. The origin of diabetes has been thought to be associated with a degenerescence, or an organic or functional alteration of the pneumogastric nerves; and it appears from observations made on diabetic patients that the first manifestation of the disease is preceded by gastric phenomena indicating a pathological condition of the stomach, and default or alteration of its digestive secretion. Now, as we have seen, dyspepsia and gastritis constitute an indication for the suspension of a stimulative and highly nitrogenous diet; and it is probable that the adoption of treatment directed on this principle in the *early* stage of the morbid condition, would suffice, particularly in cases not hereditary in origin, to prevent serious results, although it could not be hoped by such means to cure the disease in an advanced state. But when already sugar exists in large quantities in the urine, can a cure be expected by means of the exclusive use of flesh-food? No; whatever may be the course adopted, the patient will die of his complaint sooner or later. Diabetes, once passed into the cachectic stage, resembles all other cachectic conditions, and it is only in the initial stages of organic disease that science can really efficaciously interfere. To prevent the manifestation of the diathesis, or to arrest it before it becomes cachexia, these are the real functions of medicine. It is powerless to arrest a process of death already half accomplished. But, if called upon too late to treat the preliminary symptoms ; if our aid be sought when already the ingestion of farinaceous food and fruits would be injurious and even directly dangerous, ought we, from a purely medical point of view, to advise the use of lean flesh-meat, after the old classic example? No again, for only recently 'a more excellent way' has been provided by the researches and experience of Dr. Donkin, and by others who have followed his theory and practice. The diabetic patient dies of inanition; he must therefore be nourished by some form of food which is able to resist the morbid action of the liver. This desideratum appears to have been found by Dr. Donkin, and it consists of skimmed milk. He reports several cases of recovery obtained by means of its exclusive use, in a few of which the disease had already made no inconsiderable progress. Dr. Donkin demonstrates that fatty albuminous matters are always incapable of being assimilated in advanced diabetes, but that lactose and the caseine of milk deprived of its creamy part are not subject to pathological alteration. Repeated experience, he says, has convinced him by conclusive proof that the sugar, having, under a regimen of skimmed milk totally disappeared from the urine, will show itself afresh immediately after the ingestion of either *flesh-meat* or cream. The nutritive principles of skimmed milk arc lactose and caseine. Caseine, itself a nitrogenised substance, is much less apt to be converted into sugar than any other aliment of the same nature. Lactose never lends itself to the action of diabetes. Those who, with Dr. Davy, think that lactose must be injurious to diabetic patients, because it constitutes a form of sugar, are not aware of its real characteristics. The chemical properties and physiological relations of lactose differ entirely from diabetic sugar, and from every other form of glucose.

It does not undergo alcoholic fermentation; but its lactic fermentation takes place in the stomach in the presence of caseine. The amelioration of the health, the restoration of the forces, and the fact that the sugar disappears from the urine under Dr. Donkin's regimen, suffice to prove that the constituent elements of skimmed milk are well assimilated by diabetic patients. The painful symptoms and the weakness begin to pass away almost directly after the institution of the treatment; and in ordinary cases the sugar disappears from the urine after about two weeks' observance of Dr. Donkin's regimen ; and in more refractory cases, after about six weeks'. *(1)* Abstinence from flesh-food has also been found an extremely successful measure in dealing with the terrible complaint called *epilepsy*. Many theories have from time to time been suggested in explanation of the source and rationale of epileptic seizures, and of these the most seductive appears to be the recently formulated hypothesis of Dr. Hughlings-Jackson, who regards the attack as the result of nervous irritability suddenly exploded, so to speak, by an agency acting either from within or without the system, and, as by an instantaneous electric discharge, occasioning the cry, the fall, and accompanying characteristic phenomena of the disease. The fact that no lesion of other than accidental nature is found in the brains of epileptic patients, even when they have succumbed in the midst of an attack, seems evidence that the disease is of a functional and not of an organic nature; and experience has amply demonstrated that the nervous disturbance is liable to occur as the result of any exciting or stimulating action in the system. Regard for actual facts, as well as inductive reasoning, leads to the conviction that epilepsy, and its kindred disorders usually classed under the wide-reaching term 'hysteria,' ought to be treated by an absolute privation of all stimulating foods and drinks, and a persistent dietary of the farinacea, milk, fruits, and the more easily digestible vegetables, avoiding those of the 'stringy' or fibrous order.

Dr. North (U.S.) relates the case of a brother physician, who, being subject to severe attacks of epilepsy, adopted a regimen excluding all fish, flesh, and fowl for two years and a half, and during that time remained free from any attack. Dr. Hayward (U.S.) gives, in his lectures, the case of a young man who, suffering habitually from severe epilepsy, was persuaded to try a vegetable diet, and was very shortly relieved of his malady. Some time afterwards he ate freely of flesh-meat at a convivial dinner, and was immediately thrown into a violent attack. A strict adherence to a mild diet again brought immunity from seizures.

Dr. Cheyne also records a remarkable cure of epilepsy in the case of Dr. Taylor, who was for a long time dreadfully afflicted with this complaint He consulted all the most eminent of his medical *confrères* in and about London, but obtained no relief. At last it occurred to him to discontinue the use of all animal meats, and in the course of a year or two he was, by this regimen, completely cured of the disorder.

Only last year the following interesting observations on cases of the same complaint were published by Dr. George Lade: –

'Miss A— aged twenty-three, had suffered for nearly two years from slight epileptic attacks, accompanied by some uterine and hysterical symptoms, when she was brought to me for advice. The epileptic seizures occurred about once a week, sometimes oftener, mostly in the early part of the day. I prescribed such remedies as appeared to me to be indicated, and changed them from time to time as occasion, or as disappointment at their inaction, demanded; but eighteen months persistent pursuance of the treatment failed to effect any notable impression upon the features of the case. I then decided to abandon all medicines, and to try what a complete change of diet would do. I advised the patient to discontinue the use of fish and animal food, and to live entirely upon fruits and vegetables, with a moderate allowance of butter, eggs, and milk. For breakfast I suggested fruit, oatmeal porridge, bread and milk; for dinner, vegetables, fruit, brown bread, and farinaceous puddings; for supper a similar fare to that of breakfast; no beverage but water or milk-and-water. A very decided improvement was manifested in a few weeks, and went on steadily until the patient was considered cured. The dietetic treatment was adopted in October 1876, and at this date, November 10, 1877, I am assured that the patient has continued free from all epileptic symptoms for nearly five months. . . . Whether she continues to enjoy immunity from her late trouble, and still further improve in her general health, remains to be seen; but, be the result what it may, she declares she is fully resolved to adhere to the plain and unstimulating dietary, which she finds both agreeable and satisfying.

'I lately placed a young man, suffering in a similar way, upon a vegetable diet, and six weeks afterwards I was informed that the attacks were less frequent.'

Before quitting this part of our subject a few words should be said with regard to the disastrous influence exercised directly and indirectly by the use of animal food on all forms of *disease of the liver*. Nothing is commoner to witness than attacks of catarrhal icterus, or active liver congestion, in great meat-eaters; and we know that catarrh of the biliary passages brings about hepatic colics by directly causing decomposition of the cholate of soda contained in the bile, and thereby precipitating the cholesterine, which forms the greater part of the pathologic concretions known as gall-stones. The more or less grave affections of the liver, from which so many Europeans suffer in India, China, etc., are due quite as much to the stimulating and over-nitrogenised character of their diet, as to the influence of climate.

It is necessary to allude only to the treatment of *scurvy*.

Strabo is the first author who mentions this disease, which appears to have broken out for the first time in his knowledge during the Roman decadence – a fact in itself significative. The classic treatment in all cases of scorbutic manifestations, whether sporadic or epidemic, consists, as everybody knows, in the administration of fresh fruits and vegetables.

It would be a never-ending task to cite all the instances at my command of various cases of cure or of amelioration of disease and morbid diatheses of all kinds by the use of a vegetable and milk regimen. Perhaps, in concluding this portion of my work it may be well to in. form my readers that I present in my own person a sufficiently striking example of the beneficial effects of the Pythagorean system of diet, to which, indeed, I doubt not that I owe my life, my health, and the vital force I continue to enjoy. While occupied in a laborious six years' study of my profession at the *École de Médicine* of Paris, I overcame many obstacles and trials, physical and moral, rendered specially hard by the artificial disabilities of my sex, and by a variety of personal circumstances. Indeed the difficulties in my case were such as would, I believe, have proved insurmountable to most persons even of robust health and physique. I, moreover, am not only burdened with an hereditary tendency to phthisis, but have been actually treated for a somewhat severe manifestation of the disease, and am, besides, of an extremely sensitive and nervous temperament. That under all these adverse conditions I have been enabled to attain satisfactorily the end of my student's course, I owe probably in great part to the simple, pure, and unexciting diet which for a period of ten years I have uninterruptedly maintained.

In the "*Univers Illustré*" of March 26, 1876, Dr. Decaisne, writing on the subject of Lenten abstinence, affirms that many maladies are attributable to the abuse of flesh-food, and to the deplorable habits of diet to which parents usually accustom their children. Quoting Pére Debreyne, physician to La Grande-Trappe, he states that the regimen of the Trappist monks, erroneously believed to be detrimental to health and longevity, is, on the contrary, most beneficial in its effects. During a period of twenty-seven years, he has not, in this community, met with a single case of apoplexy, aneurism, dropsy, gout, gravel, or cancer. Cholera has never entered any house of the Order, even when the disease was making great ravages in the immediate vicinity of the monastery. It is notorious that no epidemic ever crosses the Trappist threshold. . . . 'Is not this calm and peaceful life,' continues Dr. Decaisne,' a most striking condemnation of our sensuality, of our intemperance, our disorders, and our passions, which destroy in us so often the very principles of life?'

And the hygienist Fonssagrives, of Montpellier, writes as follows, on the same subject: –

'Are not our peasants of Corréze and Bretagne, Pythagoreans, of necessity, though not of conviction? And is their health less robust than that of their town compatriots, who, close by, gorge themselves with flesh-meat? . . . . 'I have studied the effects of this Pythagorean method of life upon the Trappists, and found them to enjoy good health and uncommon length of life.' *(1)*

With regard to *epidemic* infection, innumerable statistics exist to prove the immunity from such visitations enjoyed by habitual abstainers from flesh and its almost invariable accompaniment, fermented drink. Among many similar examples, we find the case of Dr. Rush, cited in the 'Medical and Surgical Journal' of Edinburgh. This gentleman, during a frightful epidemic of yellow fever in Philadelphia, preserved his health and energy unimpaired by confining himself to diet consisting of vegetables, grain, and milk, excluding animal flesh in every shape.

Nothing is more remarkable, from this point of view, than the experience of the famous hygienist Sylvester Graham, who, during the New York visitation of cholera in the year 1832, persuaded a considerable number of the citizens – in direct opposition to general medical advice – to abstain rigorously from all flesh-meats and alcoholic drinks, and to restrict themselves entirely to a vegetable diet. 'It is,' says Mr. Graham, 'an important fact that of all who followed the prescribed regimen, not one fell a victim to the disease, and very few had the slightest symptoms of an attack.'

Drs. Pollard, Rees, and Tappan, who also, during the same epidemic, prescribed a similar dietary for their clients, had the satisfaction to see all of them, without exception, preserve excellent health in the midst of the universal suffering and death which surrounded them. *(2)*

FOOTNOTES
(75:1) Chrisitison.

(76:1) The Jews, according to Dr. Richardson, appear to enjoy remarkably fine and regular health; the duration of life among them exceeds by a fourth or fifth that of every European nation.

(78:1) Dr. Abernethy, the celebrated Scotch surgeon of the last century, gave it as his opinion that all 'animal substances become changed in the economy into a putrid, abominable, and acrid stimulus.' Whether this view be scientifically correct or not, it is incontestable that excrements resulting from the ordinary mixed diet have a highly offensive factor which, in the case of a purely vegetable alimentation, becomes a hardly perceptible odour. It may be added that the strength of this effluvium increases with the amount of animal food ingested. The lame remark, other things being equal, applies to the breath. How often have I immediately diagnosed a great eater of flesh by no other sign than the odour of the exhalation of his lungs!

(79:1) Treatise on Food.

(80:1) Dr. Austin Flint *(Experiments and Reflections upon Animal Heat)* thinks that if the excessive heat of fever be partly due to excessive oxydation of hydrogen, the exhaustion and loss of substance thus caused might be moderated by the ingestion of hydrogen under the form of fatty, starchy, and sugary matters.

(81:1) Andral and Gavarret.

(82 :1) Dr. Rendu's Etudes des Nephrites Chroniques,1880.

(83:1) Claude Bernard's experiments on himself.

(83:2) Dr. Prout goes still further; he likens the lithiac diathesis to that of scrofula, and alleges that both are the expression of the presence in excess, or of the lack of power to assimilate, the nitrogenous element. According to him, gouty concretions are but a modification of phthisic tubercle.

(87:1) On the Relation between Diabetes and Food, and its application in the Treatment of the Disease by Arthur Scott Donkin, M.D., 1875.

(92:1) Diet.

(92:2) Smith's Fruits and Farinacea.

13. ECONOMICAL CONSIDERATION

We now approach a new aspect of our many-sided subject, an aspect certainly not less interesting than those already examined, and affecting on one hand the Nation, on the other the Individual. I speak of Economy.

Let us see first how it affects the Nation.

In the face of the ever rapidly increasing tide of population, a population which doubles its numbers every fifty-six years, no questions can be of greater interest to the political economist than those relating to the nature and cost of the national food-supply. Mr. Greg in his 'Enigmas of Life' makes the following observations, which, although involving the extreme hypothesis of a wholly carnivorous diet as opposed to one wholly graminivorous, are nevertheless thoroughly sensible and to the purpose: –

'There is one mode in which the amount of human existence sustainable on a given area, and therefore throughout the chief portion of the habitable globe, may be almost indefinitely increased, *i.e. by a substitution of vegetable for animal food.* A given acreage of wheat will feed at least ten times as many men as the same acreage employed in growing mutton. It is usually calculated that the consumption of wheat by an adult is about one quarter per annum, and we know that good land produces four quarters. Let us even assume that a man living on grain would require two quarters a year; still one acre would support two men. But a man living on (flesh) meat would need three pounds a day, and it is considered a liberal calculation if an acre spent in grazing sheep and cattle yields in mutton or beef more than fifty pounds on an average – the best farmer in Norfolk having averaged ninety pounds; but a great majority of farms in Great Britain only reach twenty pounds. On these data, it would require twenty-two acres of pastureland to sustain one adult person living on meat (alone). It is obvious that in view of the adoption of vegetable diet, there lies the indication of a vast possible increase in the population sustainable on a given area.'

Reflections such as these had begun to press on the minds of politicians more than a century ago, about which time we find the well-known theological essayist Dr. Paley, writing thus in his 'Principles of Moral and Political Philosophy:' –

'So far as the state of population is governed and limited by the quantity of provision, perhaps there is no single cause that affects it so powerfully as the kind and quality of food which chance or usage hath introduced into a country. In England, notwithstanding the produce of the soil has been of late considerably increased by the enclosure of wastes, and the adoption, in many places, of a more successful husbandry, yet we do not observe a corresponding addition to the number of inhabitants, the reason of which appears to me to be the more general consumption of animal food amongst us. Many ranks of people whose ordinary diet was, in the last century, prepared almost entirely from milk, roots, and vegetables, now require every day a considerable portion of the flesh of animals. *Have a great part of the richest lands of the country are converted to pasturage.* Much also of the bread-corn, which went directly to the nourishment of human bodies, now only contributes to it by fattening the flesh of sheep and oxen. *The mass and volume of provisions are hereby diminished*; and what is gained in the amelioration of the soil is lost in the quality of the produce. This consideration teaches us that tillage, as an object of national care and encouragement, is universally preferable to pasturage, because the kind of provision which it yields goes much farther in the sustentation of human life. Tillage is Also recommended by this additional advantage, that it *affords employment to a much more numerous peasantry.* . . . If we measure the quantity of provision by the number of human bodies it will support in due health and vigour, this quantity, the extent and quality of the soil from which it is raised being given, will depend greatly upon the *kind*. For instance, a piece of ground capable of supplying animal food sufficient for the subsistence of ten persons, *would sustain at least the double of (hat number with grain, roots, and milk!*

A paper entitled '*Food Thrift*,' from the pen of Dr. Richardson in '*Modern Thought*' for July 1880, contains the following words: –

'Under a mere bagatelle of pressure, less man such an extreme pressure as is above suggested (hostile blockade), England would in a short time be convulsed politically, not from actual deficiency of supply, but from the difference of ability on the part of the consumers to lay by stores of supply. A sharp demand, a panic, the few rich would practically buy up the multitudinous poor, and then, when the multitude hungered, or even fancied it hungered, would come the crash. . . . If produce be shared unequally and savagely, some must die of want by necessity. Shared equally and with love, none need die of want anywhere, neither in the coldest nor most unfruitful region, except by accident or self-disregard.' Speaking of emigration, Dr. Richardson adds: – 'It is the fittest for work and for earning who leave our shores – the unfittest for work, the luxurious, and the least powerful remain. Thus the drain on the first processes of national permanent prosperity is that which is opened by emigration, and is that which is exhausting the heart of the Commonwealth. . . . We really ought to consider the question of utilising, on a large scale, all vegetables which, in nutrient value, stand above animal products. We have also to learn, as a first truth, the truth that the oftener we go to the vegetable world for our food, the oftener we go to the first, and, therefore, to the cheapest source of supply. The commonly accepted notion that when we eat animal flesh we are eating food at its prime source cannot be too speedily dissipated, or too speedily replaced by the knowledge that there is no primitive form of food – albuminous, starchy, osseous – in the animal world itself, and that all the processes of catching an inferior animal, or of breeding it, rearing it, keeping it, dressing it, and selling it, mean no more nor less than entirely additional expenditure throughout for bringing into what we have been taught to consider an acceptable form of food the veritable food which the animal itself found, without any such preparation, in the vegetable world.'

Addressing the electors of Salford on February 20, 1879, Mr. Arthur Arnold said: –

'The green curtain which our land system has encouraged Nature to draw over the depopulation of Ireland is now advancing from the west towards the east of England. Where the ploughman was wont to whistle over agriculture, the beast grazes, requiring nearly three acres of pasture to produce the quantity of meat which one acre would yield to suitable tillage.'

The old saying, 'Where God sends mouths he sends food,' is no mere superstitious pretext for recklessness. By obeying the wholesome dictates of Nature, and leading in all particulars natural lives, we shall find the earth yielding an abundance of all we require for the sustenance of our offspring. Each child means not only a life to be supported, but also a pair of hands to till the ground, and each pair of hands can produce in grain more than is needed for the owner's support It is thus that in a better distribution of the soil rather than in the practice of 'Malthusianism,' the desired reformation ought to be sought. So far from siding with the chilling and sordid doctrines advocated under this name, there is surely something noble in that faith in Nature's capacity which prompts our race to increase and multiply upon the earth, trusting to the response which that earth is ready to yield to industrious toil. The essential selfishness of Malthusianism is one of the strongest objections that can be urged against its practice. By restricting the production of offspring in the most highly developed races, or in the most highly cultivated families of any race, the future of the world is virtually abandoned to the lowest types, and these would thus be enabled before long completely to outnumber and suppress the higher. The energy which prompts us to multiply is but part of the same *vis viva* which leads us to appropriate and colonise every available spot of the earth's surface. Had the doctrines of Malthus been adopted by Britons during the last three centuries, the whole continent of America might at this moment have been in the hands of people such as that now occupying its central States, a people which must be reckoned among the least worthy of those claiming to be civilised. Professor Newman, writing in '*Fraser's Magazine*,' says: –

'That by living on vegetable food, a larger population might be supported, Malthus was aware. It does not seem to have occurred to him to remark, that only by consenting to become chiefly vegetarian has any nation become populous; that while the population is sparse, nations have been comparatively barbarous ; and that the adoption of vegetarian diet has been one condition of civilisation and power. It is calculated, that to produce the same quantity of human food (on a low average) as a *cultivated* acre will yield, three or four acres of glaring land are needed for flesh-meat; and if the most profitable crop be selected for comparison, six or seven acres is nearer the truth. . . . We are told that England is over-peopled; we ask, "What is the proof?" It is replied, "There is constant pressing distress." It is wonderful that this seems to any one a satisfactory reply. If the population were at once cut down to what it was when Malthus's first edition appeared, is it certain that there would be no such distress? Nay, there was then such poverty that he assumed the country over-peopled. Mere want and suffering, however constant, can never prove that there is *too much population*; to assume that it does is a perpetual fallacy of our economists. *Too much vice, too much bad law,* causing waste and disease, will infallibly produce suffering and pauperism, whatever the natural abundance and natural advantages for crops. In 1871 it was computed that the yearly destruction of grain to produce beer and spirits was such as would produce 1,050 million four-pound loaves; besides this 61,792 acres of the best land are used for growing hops. Thus, by ceasing to drink beer and spirits, there would be a great increase to the available human food, to say nothing of the vast *over-eating* and *waste* almost universal in our rich towns. *(1)* What is more important still – if this one vice of drunkenness were cut off, a prodigious mass of misery would be removed, out of which spring pauperism and new vice; the greater part of violent crime would vanish, and the vast waste of labour occasioned . . . would be saved No doubt when the people are kept from the land, they cannot get food out of it. . . . but for that very reason, the question "Is the land over-peopled ?" has never been put to any real test at all.'

According to Lance, Middleton, Rawson, Breton, and other authorities, the estimated produce of an acre of land in various kinds (excluding of course special considerations with regard to soil, climate, season, etc.) is the following: –

Produce	Per Year Lbs.	Per Day
Mutton *(1)*	228	10
Beef *(1)*	182 1/2	8 lbs
Wheat *(2)*	1,680	4 1/2
Barley	1,800	5
Oats	2,300	6
Peas	1,650	4 1/2
Beans	1,800	5s
Indian corn (maize)	3,120	8 1/2
Rice	4,565	12 1/2
Potatoes	20,160	55
Parsnips	26,880	74
Carrots	33,600	92
Yams	40,000	110
Turnips	56,000	154
Beets	75,000	205

If we suppose a third of the whole extent of land at our disposal consecrated to the production of the cereals, and of such leguminous plants as peas, beans, etc.; a third to that of potatoes, beets, turnips (tubers and roots), and the remaining third to the culture of fruits, forests, and pasturage for the rearing of oxen, cows, sheep, etc., whose labour, milk, and wool would be utilised, we should, under such conditions, be able to support, on the same area, a population many times greater than the present.

There is a branch of fanning which, in this country, does not receive half the attention it deserves. I refer to the cultivation of orchards and fruit-gardens. If the land in England were cultivated more like a garden, our population would be fully and profitably employed, and we should want but little emigration and foreign supplies. Many clay soils which are not remunerative under a corn crop, would be useful to their owners, and valuable to the country, if planted with apple, pear, or plum trees. And, with regard to the cost of building pits and forcing-houses for the rearing of less hardy fruits – a proceeding which the exigencies of our climate would necessitate – the original outlay requisite on such structures and stocking would not exceed, if indeed it would equal, the sums of money risked annually upon the purchase and breeding of cattle, constantly subject to all manner of epidemics and diseases. Moreover, it may not be generally known, that, on the plea of assisting food supply, Parliament has been pleased to help private individuals at the public expense. In 1861 inspectors were appointed to aid in the promotion and extension of the Scotch salmon fisheries, and this aid, originally enacted for three years, has been annually renewed to the fishery owners by successive Governments. Why should not Parliament be equally kind to fruit-growers and market-gardeners on the ground of concern for the national food supply?' In the face of the present agricultural depression,' says the 'Nottingham Evening Post,' 'farmers might very advantageously direct their attention to planting waste pieces of land with fruit trees. Though the return for money expenditure in that way is not immediate, it is sure, if the work is properly done. There is no doubt that were more public attention directed to this question, a great impetus would be given to the cultivation of fruit; not only would there be more trees planted, but the extra yield would be more than proportionately increased, owing to improved methods of cultivation. The home food supply would be considerably greater, and the increase would be of that kind of food which has an especially beneficial effect on the human frame. The true wealth of our country would be augmented, and the condition of those engaged in the most wholesome and primary of English home industries would be improved. Local flower and horticultural shows do much towards the encouragement of horticulture and fruit culture, but they have a very different effect from that which would follow the appointment of a public inspector. He who competes at a show aims at *producing fine* fruit and vegetables, and it is for these that he has prizes offered him. No direct encouragement is thus offered to the occupier of waste plots of ground and hedge-rows to plant them with fruit trees. There would be a far better chance of such a desirable end being brought about if Government were to take the matter in hand. This is not a political matter, but an economical one. It is one which must in time receive more public attention; and, in the meantime, those who believe with us will do well to exert themselves individually to promote the fruit-growing capacities of the country.'

With regard to the utilisation of land lying waste and idle in and about towns or hamlets, it has been suggested that the 'labour test' might be applied in this direction with useful results, and that paupers, in return for the relief afforded them out of the public rates, might be employed advantageously in many districts as drainers, tillers, and agriculturists; a measure which would not only lead to increase in the value of the wastes so utilised, but would conduce also in no small degree to sanitary improvement, by draining off stagnant pools, appropriating to purposes of manure innumerable rubbish heaps, rendering the general atmosphere purer, and ridding the country of some of its worst nuisances.

We have seen, thus briefly, in what manner the economical question affects the country and the nation. Let us now inquire how it affects the Individual.

According to Dr. Lyon Playfair, F.R.S., C.B., who for several years directed a series of official investigations on the subject of military radons in England, France, Prussia, and Austria, an adult man in good health requires daily four ounces of proteinaceous substances, and at least ten and a half ounces daily of dynamic substances (hydro-carbons and carbo-hydrates). In order to obtain this proportion of proteinaceous matter it would be necessary to consume *weekly*: –

Price (about)

			s.	d.
147 ounces of		butcher's meat	6	1
or 93	"	cheese	3	0
or 341	"	ordinary white bread	2	8
or 175	"	oatmeal	1	4
or 127	"	dried peas	1	2

In order to obtain the necessary proportion of dynamic or caloric-forming substance, it would be necessary to consume *weekly*: –

Price (about)

			s.	d.
416 ounces of butcher's		meat	17	4
or 224	,,	cheese	7	0
or 298	,,	ordinary bread	2	3
or 616	,,	potatoes	2	9
or 221	,,	dried peas	11	0
or 183	,,	oatmeal	1	0

It will be seen, according to these tables, that the same elements of nutrition are furnished by bread, cheese, oat-meal, and peas at a price invariably less than half that of butcher's meat, and that, if the cheese be excepted, the difference of cost is much more remarkable.

Dr. Edward Smith, F.R.S., who, in 1864, under the direction of the Government, conducted certain inquiries into the kind and quantity of food in use among the poor classes, showed that at the same price – taking a penny as unit – a man may have: –

	Grains of Carbon	Grains of Nitrogen
Bread	1450	66
Barley	2500	93
Oat-meal	1513	75
Wheat-meal	1330	60
Rice	1380	35
Maize	2800	121
Peas	1830	170
Milk	873	87
Beef	320	23
Mutton	415	20
Pork	483	18
Ham	510	12

We have then in favour of a vegetable dietary a *quadruple* economy.

In a paper read before the Manchester Statistical Society, by Mr. W. Hoyle, the waste caused by the prevailing dietetic habits of the population was thus epitomised: –

'There is not only much loss and waste by defective agriculture and by waste of sewage, but also by an injudicious use of food. . . . It is proved that a shilling's worth of flour or oatmeal, as well as fruit and other vegetable goods, will give as much nourishment as five shillings' worth of flesh. . . . and if we assume that, on the average, the six million families of the United Kingdom reduced their consumption of animal food by only one pound a week, it would give a saving of ten or twelve million pounds sterling per annum.'

Elsewhere the same statistician observes that it is possible to buy in vegetable food five times the quantity of nutritive matter obtainable for the same price in animal food, and that the sum necessary to support yearly a single person living on the ordinary mixed fare would suffice to sustain at least three or four vegetarians.

The average results of all these calculations, which it would be easy but useless to multiply by further references, and the examination of the comparative value of animal and vegetable products, whether wholesale or retail, may be thus resumed: –

1. A given area of ground, consecrated to the culture of corn, vegetables, and fruit, and to pasturage sufficient to meet the needs of a non-flesh-eating people, would yield provision capable of sustaining a population about six times greater than the same area as at present distributed.

2. A vegetable dietary, to which even cheese, butter, and milk are added, costs per head three or four times less than a mixed dietary of flesh and vegetables.

Hence the economy of *land*, the economy of *expense*, and consequently both national and private wealth and prosperity would be enormously increased by a return to the dietetic habits indicated as natural to man by his physical structure and by his moral instincts. And indeed we feel it impossible to insist too strongly on the value and importance of these economical considerations when we reflect on the misery and suffering which exist everywhere, especially in great cities. The extent and grossness of the ignorance of the poor on the subject of the physiological relation and chemical value of foods cannot be gauged; it is equalled only by their general obstinacy and unwillingness to be instructed on the subject Yet there lies before them a Way to Paradise, simple enough and straight enough for all to take – a way by following which the poor might all attain health, happiness, ease, and the comfort of rearing children without dread of famine, vice, or slavery.

FOOTNOTES

(98:1) We have already observed that kreophagy and alcoholism are, so to speak, inseparable companions, whose steps keep pace one with the other.

(99:1) These are Middleton's statements. In England the estimate of Mr. Greg – less than one half the above – is probably more correct.

(99:2) Good land, especially under spade husbandry, will produce a great deal more.

14. OVER-BREEDING

If it be asked, 'What then is to become of all the animals? Shall we not be overrun by them?' the answer to such questions is not far to seek. Cease to breed beasts for purposes of food. Nature will know how to right herself and recover the equilibrium which man has violated. The breeding of cattle and game is far in excess of nature. These creatures are multiplied intentionally by human intervention, by selection, by importation, and by all imaginable contrivances. It must, however, be borne in mind that, with the increase of culture and tillage which is advocated by the reformed system, a large number of oxen would be required to aid in agricultural labour – their ancient and legitimate service. As for rabbits, hares, and feathered game, everyone knows that these animals are maintained in excessive numbers for purposes of 'sport.' *(1)* That, for the time being, artificial habits have disturbed the just balance of nature is proved by the fact that those creatures which are not used for food by man do not increase to any appreciable, still less to any injurious, extent. Do we risk being devoured or overrun by badgers, bearers, squirrels, hedgehogs, donkeys, horses? Or of being pecked out of house and home by robins, starlings, or goldfinches? Have we not even great difficulty in obtaining horses and other beasts of burden at reasonable prices, although these creatures are never killed for food, save by a few eccentrics in Paris? Nature indeed, unless man wilfully disarrange her laws, so regulates the mutual relation of things as to prevent the undue multiplication of any one kind of animal.

Again, it is in the last degree improbable that the conversion of the world from its present habits to a purer system will be other than very gradual. Therefore those creatures which are now artificially increased will have ample time to decrease gradually in number as the demand for their flesh gradually lessens. Most of these animals, too, let us recollect, are not indigenous to our climate, but have been at a remote period imported from distant parts of the globe; the ox probably from Oriental countries, the sheep from Africa. Among our captive descendants of the wild kine there have been so many changes wrought by the hand of man as strangely to modify nature. Those enfeebled, indolent, sad-faced animals which we see in our fields and streets are a degenerate race, shaped by art and propagated merely to pamper vicious appetites. Stand awhile in any pasture and observe the sheep. He is a mere mass of flesh, supported on four small straight legs, ill-fitted for carrying such a burden. His movements are awkward and slothful, he is easily fatigued, and frequently sinks under the weight of his own corpulence. And in proportion to the degree of the transformation to which human device has subjected him and his ancestry, the creature becomes more helpless, inert, and stupid. Oxen and sheep which batten upon very fertile lands become fat and feeble to an extraordinary degree, those that lack horns being the dullest and heaviest, while those whose fleeces are longest and finest are most subject to disease.

In short, whatever changes have been wrought in these doomed and unfortunate brutes by man are entirely calculated to bring them under the same curse of disease and degradation as that which man has brought upon himself. For the truth is, as has been said by the poet Shelley, himself one of the apostles of our doctrine: –

'Man, and the other animals whom he has depraved by his dominion, are alone diseased. Wild creatures are exempt from malady, and die either by accident or from mature old age. But the domestic hog, sheep, cow, and dog are subject to an incredible variety of distempers, and, like the corruptors of their nature, have physicians who thrive upon their miseries. The supereminence of man is the supereminence of pain.'

But, while on questions of economy, distribution, and commerce, it is proper to say a word on some other points which occur in connection with the traffic in and consumption of flesh, the chief of which concern the interests of the leather and fur trades, the use of animal manure, and the practices of 'sport' and trapping.

FOOTNOTES

(105:1) Not long ago rabbits were reported to have become so scarce in Denmark that an agent of that country was commissioned to import 50,000 of these animals from France to recruit the Danish warrens.

15. THE LEATHER QUESTION

With regard to the first two considerations, we may safely rely on the time-proven axiom of commerce, that demand creates supply. If, for instance, any large section of the public should insist on having vegetable leather, the article before long would be plentiful in the market, and improvements in its manufacture would continuously be announced. That already, even in the absence of any great demand, it is in the market, is evident from the following, taken from the *'Leather Merchants' Almanac'* (1877): –

'Under the title of "Improvements in the Manufacture of Vegetable Leather" a patent has recently been obtained in this country for an invention which promises to utilise certain waste and cheap products. Fucus of several species, and laminaria are well known sea-weeds, as plentiful on the sea coast as grass in the fields, and waste textile materials of vegetable origin are in sufficient abundance to find profitable employment in the manufacture of this leather. Sheets of carded wadding are manufactured from cotton waste or from cotton itself, according to the quality required, of uniform thickness, length, and width. These sheets are then placed on polished zinc or other metal plates, and coated with a concentrated decoction of *fucus crispus* or pearl moss, or other fucus or mucilaginous lichen, or with any similar substance. The metal plates require to be kept hot in order to allow the decoction to penetrate thoroughly into the filaments of the cotton. The sheet is then dried quickly, thus giving to the surface applied to the metal plate a glazed or polished appearance, resembling the gloss of ordinary leather, and, thus prepared, it is passed between two heated cylinders or rollers perfectly polished, having a space between them according to the thickness required. Great pressure is needed to press all the filaments of cotton thoroughly together, and to render the thickness uniform. It is then coated with boiled linseed oil, and dried in the open air, or by artificial heat. When dry, a coat of thin vegetable wax is applied, and the sheet is softened by passing through heated fluted rollers; it is then passed through other polished rollers according to the quality required, either plain, morocco, embossed, glazed, or otherwise, and is next bronzed, varnished, and finished like ordinary leather. It is waterproof and easily stamped.'

A similar leather has been introduced still more recently into French commerce.

16. CRUELTY OF THE FUR-TRADE

As for the furs, they are worn rather as a luxury and ornament than as a necessity, and may easily be dispensed with, even by the most delicate, and in our northern climate, as I myself know by personal experience. Let the following short sketch of some of the horrors of the fur trade suffice to give a faint idea of the price we pay in blood and suffering for the furs which decorate our women, and what cost to human nature, which no gold can compensate, is involved by obedience to the careless whims of fashion.

'Man desires hides, horns, feathers ivory; and considers himself fully justified in satisfying these desires, however extreme or whimsical, by the destruction of life. The savage, in need of clothing and unable to manufacture woollen garments, may indeed plead the necessity of wrapping himself in furs; but can civilised man, who is well acquainted with the art of producing artificial coverings, equal if not superior to furs, advance the same plea? He must urge in justification of his killing and torturing in order to obtain furs and feathers, not his necessities, but his luxuries, whims, and caprices. It may be useful to glance at the sealskin trade as an instance in point. Unfortunately for the seal and for humanity, a method has been discovered of converting the greyish hue of its fur into a rich lustrous brown. Forthwith sealskins have become the rage, and find a ready sale at high prices. To obtain them extensive hunting expeditions are organised and conducted with an amount of cruelty which is perhaps without parallel. in all the dealings of man towards the lower animals. Seals are most readily captured at the time when they have young cubs not yet capable of following their mothers through the water. At this time they may be found upon the shores *of* certain Arctic regions in great numbers, and here accordingly they are attacked. The mother seals are stunned with blows from clubs and then flayed, often before dead, it being considered that the fur is thus obtained in a more lustrous condition. The little seals are left to perish of cold and hunger. The frightful atrocity of this system will be more fully understood if we remember that the seal stands high in the scale of animal life, and possesses a large well-developed brain and a delicate nervous system. All this cruelty is therefore perpetrated for the sake of "fashion," and to it all wearers of sealskin jackets make themselves accessory. It is true that some voices have been raised against this system, and that some attempts have been made to mitigate its horrors by legislative enactments, but there is every reason to fear that as long as the demand for sealskin continues, the supply will be obtained substantially in the manner we have sketched' *(1)*

The '*Daily Telegraph*,' in an article on the same subject, says: —

'The time chosen for the hunting is unfortunately the very period that of all others ought to be kept close. Except for a very short part of the year the seal lives to all intents and purposes on the open sea. But the female, when about to bring forth, seeks the shelter of the shore, where she suckles and watches her cubs until they are old enough to shift for themselves. At this time, wherever there are seals along the coast herds of them will be found from a quarter to half a mile inland. The proportions are very much those of a drove of deer. The main body will consist of females, each with one or two helpless little ones, while the males keep about the outskirts of the flock. . . . As soon as a herd of this kind is spied, the boats are manned, and the whole vessel's crew, armed with bludgeons and axes, starts upon a "cutting-out expedition," at the horrors of which humanity may well shudder. The only way to effectually kill a seal with completeness and despatch is by a heavy blow with a bludgeon, or a deep cut with an axe, so as either to crush or sever the nasal bones; and when the boats' crews have got ashore, an indiscriminate slaughter is commenced, the whole herd being often butchered before a single one can reach the water's edge. . . . The adult quarry is skinned with all possible haste, and as often as not with the life still in it The cubs, who lie moaning and whinnying by the side of their dams, are knocked on the head if big enough to give their fur any value, and if too small to be worth the skinning are left without even the mercy of a *coup de grâce*. Old seal-hunters tell us — and we can well believe it — that it takes a man some time *to get used* to such cruel butchery, and that the half-human wailing of the little seals, as they climb and roll about the mangled carcase of their mother, is a sound that, *until he is hardened to the work*, will make a man's sleep uneasy at night'

Yet one more quotation on this subject, the ethics of which are so homely, and so important to women, who should be, above all things, merciful.

'If there be a specially unpleasant sight,' says the '*Birmingham Town Crier*,' 'it is to see a group of dirty rascals prowling along the hedge-rows, intent on the massacre of small birds. The birds are the heralds of a better time, but their low-bred and dirty assassins seem to be the heralds of some dismal future, in which joy shall be dead, admiration impossible, and gratitude unknown. Vastly different are the dainty ladies who trip up and down our streets and turn their gloom into gaiety. These are nicely dressed, have smiling faces, wear fair colours, and are pleasant to see. . . . And yet there is one little bond of union between the fellow lurking behind the hedge-row, and the dainty lady who has just stepped out of some handsome carriage. The man has just wrung the neck of a wounded thrush, and stuffed it into his pocket to join the last shot blackbird ; and the woman has a bird's bright wing stuck on one side of her pretty hat; and on the other side a tiny humming bird, all gold, and bronze, and green, and scarlet, nods at each movement of its wearer. Yes, and we are authoritatively told that these adornments of our women are torn from the birds while yet alive, that the plumage may have its full brilliancy.

'Now women ought to know that they have literally no excuse for indulging in these barbarities. They have worn almost every object that can possibly be fastened to human dress. As a rule, whatever women wear seems to become them, and they have no excuse for seeking out strange devices, least of all for encouraging bird slaughter, out of the mere idleness of vanity, and for the sake of fashion. There is not one man on the face of this earth, who is not a knave or a fool, who will admire any woman the more because she has some slaughtered bird's plumage in her bonnet. We know that those things are mere ornament. They do not protect, they do not comfort; their sole office is to adorn, and they are literally to be ranked amongst the most brutal adornments that the depravity of bad taste has ever hung about human creatures. No woman who wears these things can know the beauty of living birds; can ever have watched them in the long spring days, or have listened to them as daylight lingers, and the air is heavy with fragrance, and glad with music. The dainty goldfinch, clad in a livery which seems as if it had been designed to unite grace with gaiety, and to show how great glory can dwell with the smallest of this earth, asks but a few thistle seeds to live on. His ways are charming, his colours are delightful, his music is heavenly, and he is fast disappearing that women's hats may be stuck over with wings torn from his living body. So we might go through the catalogue, for no bird is sacred from the harpies who in the secret dens of fashion dress out their dolls and paint their idols, – idols as of old that crave for life, and are as of old to be satisfied only with living sacrifices.

'A little thought only is wanted; a little reflection, and the hand of the bird-assassin would be stayed, and his hideous trade ended. Or is the example of our "highest" too strong for us who are in lowly places? Has the taint of Hurlingham spread over the whole nation? Is it too late for the conscience of an outraged humanity to rise against that tyranny of fashion which daily seeks to stain its sports more deeply with blood, and to adorn its women with the spoils of cruelty and pain?'

FOOTNOTES

(110:1) American Journal, 1877.

17. THE MANURE QUESTION

Next, with regard to the question sometimes asked, how the soil is to be manured for crops, if any considerable decrease should take place in the numbers of our cattle. Professor Laws, who has made the study of manures the work of his life, and who is the recognised authority on this question all over the world, has written as follows: –

'In all cases where artificial food is employed, or where the consumption of food is not attended with profit, it is better to restore the superabundance of green crops directly to the soil for the after-growth of corn, than to pass it through the stomachs of animals. There is no magical property in the black mass called dung which does not exist in the food, and the passage of straw or turnips through the viscera of an animal, so far from adding to the value of these substances used as manure, abstracts a large proportion of their valuable elements.'

'It may be further pointed out,' says a correspondent of the 'Dietetic Reformer,' commenting on the above extract, 'that Mr. Smith, the successful farmer of Woolston, has never put a barrowful of manure on his land in his life. He ploughs deeply in the autumn, and allows the air to manure the ground during the winter, before sowing in the spring.'

18. SPORT

Still more closely connected with the *rationale* of systematic kreophagy are the ethics, traditions, and achievements of 'sport.'

In his highest development man is not a hunter, but a gardener. The spirit of the Garden is incompatible with that of the Chase, and the inevitable tendency of moral, intellectual, and aesthetic progress is to eradicate in man the desire to kill and to torment. The destruction of life for mere destruction's sake has never been, and cannot be, a source of pleasure to any civilised human being; and, where such destruction is necessary, as in the clearing of jungle-lands and other districts infested by carnivora, poisonous reptiles, and vermin, the work of extermination should be undertaken rather as a duty than as a pastime, precisely as righteous war is undertaken by the hero, being neither shunned for selfish motives, nor compromised with for convenience or comfort's sake, but intrepidly and conscientiously performed in the spirit of the redeemer. For the true man is the redeemer, not the tyrant of the earth.

Moved, perhaps, by such sentiments as these, Montaigne, the celebrated French essayist of the sixteenth century, who has aptly been called 'the modern Plutarch,' expresses himself thus on the subject of the chase, in his days as popular as now: –

'For my part I have never been able to see, without displeasure, an innocent and defenceless animal, from whom we receive no offence or harm, pursued and slaughtered. And when a deer, as commonly happens, finding herself without breath and strength, without other resource, throws herself down and surrenders, as it were, to her pursuers, begging for mercy by her tears,

Questuque cruentus
Atque imploranti similis,' *(1)*
this has always appeared to me a very sad spectacle.'

Yet so little way with the mass of people has been made by the generous and manly spirit thus expressed, during a period of more than two centuries, that week after week in the 'sporting season' our newspapers record the wholesale slaughter of hares, pheasants, grouse, and other animals in the preserves of some illustrious member of the Upper House; and it is written for our learning that his Royal Highness or his ducal grace 'bagged,' like any poulterer, so many head of game. At Hurlingham and elsewhere, where the 'nobility' (save the mark!) of the country accustom themselves to do butcher's work on an incredible number of tame and defenceless pigeons, it is forbidden by the laws of sport to aim twice at the same bird If, therefore, the shooter should not be sufficiently dexterous to kill his victim at first fire, the wretched bird falls wounded on the grass, and pants away its life as best it may. And while the poor dead and dying doves drop bleeding at their feet, creatures with the forms and the faces of women sit by in gala attire, laughing, chattering, and smiling their sweetest on the slaughterers.

Then we have the battues, which are perhaps even more horrible and savage in their details than the pigeon 'sport,' and these, too, are attended by ladies. Long since the voice of this country condemned bear-baiting, bull-fighting, and the sport of the cockpit. But the spirit of these barbarous games still survives at Hurlingham and in the park-preserves of many a noble peer.

One word in conclusion on the subject of trapping. Farmers, owners of rabbit-warrens, gardeners, bailiffs of large properties, and others are in the daily habit of using for the destruction of ground vermin, gins so ingeniously and hideously cruel that one can hardly read the description of them without a shudder. These gins are constructed with a spring which snaps violently on the animal's leg, bruising, cutting, and often breaking it, and very often completely separating the softer parts of the limb from the bone. All the rabbits I have seen taken from these traps had the feet more than half severed, and the wounds inflamed by a struggle of many hours' duration; for the creatures are generally caught in the gins overnight, and throughout the long interval which supervenes until the keeper makes his morning rounds, they hang torn, lacerated, and terrified on the teeth of the vice, beating and rending their wounds in their frantic efforts to escape. 'It is a grim reflection,' as the *'Lancet'* well observes, 'that all this suffering is inflicted with no sufficient object The only rational explanation of the cruelty seems to be that those who set traps of this class in their grounds are unaware of the extent to which such engines maim and agonise the creatures caught in them. It would in truth be difficult to exaggerate the suffering they entail.'

As for the bird-traps, the captive taken in these is seized generally by the feet and hangs head downwards for four or five days, till it dies of starvation or exhaustion from struggling.

These are matters which might be separately and directly dealt with by the Legislature. They are named here only because they bear a family relation and likeness to that class of barbarisms, wastes, and blunders, of which the shambles, the chase, the battue, and the vivisector's laboratory are characteristic types, and whose spirit is inherently antagonistic to the needs, intuition, and progress of civilised humanity.

FOOTNOTES

(115:1) 'With plaintive cries, all covered with blood, and in the attitude of a suppliant.' – Virgil's *Aeneis*, viii.

19. RECAPITULATION

It has now been shown – briefly indeed, but I trust sufficiently – what support for the system advocated in these pages is derived from the facts of comparative anatomy, physiology, history, chemistry, and political and social economy; what corroboration for its doctrines is furnished by the actual experience of modern nations and communities, by the testimony of experimental medicine, and by the consideration of the moral duties we owe to our own kind and to the races below us. In regard to this last point, it must be remembered, no social or philosophical system is scientific and complete which omits from its definition of humanity the moral nature, since it is precisely the development of the sentiments – honour, love, justice, generosity – which distinguishes the human being from the brute, the civilised man from the savage and the criminal.

And if, for the vindication of the views advanced in these pages it be necessary or helpful to adduce authority, they have as advocates such a mighty array of names ancient and modern as no other school which the world has yet seen can boast To these illustrious names of men who have thought as I think, and whose disciple no one need be ashamed to be, I make appeal; to Pythagoras and Gautama Buddha, to Socrates, Seneca, and Plutarch, to Porphyry, and Apollonius of Tyana, to Origen, Chrysostom, and Francis Assisi, to Gassendi, Gleizes, and Shelley – in short, to all the most serious and luminous minds of the ancient and modem world.

For with all these the first essential step towards perfectionment, whether of the individual or of the community, was so to regulate life that its sustenance should involve no shock to the moral conscience.

The doctrine, which is that of the modern school of abstainers from flesh, was that of the Magi who initiated Daniel; of the Therapeuts, who drew their origin and their knowledge from Egyptian adepts; of the Buddhists, an expression of whose beautiful teaching is prefixed to this essay; of the Nazarites, who counted Jesus among their number; of the Essenes, who produced his friend and companion, John the Baptist; of the Ebionites and Recluses; of the exponents of the Christian 'Gnosis,' who kept alive and bequeathed to us through the Neo-Platonists that spirit of understanding, that 'seeing eye' and 'hearing ear' possible only in their completeness to men of pure heart and life.

In extolling this pure heart, in advocating this clean and blameless life, in indicating this perfect way, we imitate the illuminati of all ages. May those who are as yet unable wholly to endorse their practice and ours, pardon at least the love which inspires a project of emancipation from the tyranny of disease, luxury, injustice, poverty, and melancholy, which, under the present system, have attained such a height as to render existence well-nigh insupportable!

20. CONCLUSION

Thus, in the recoil from a pseudo-civilisation, the mind reverts for the principles of a true civilisation to times long past; and this treatise, whose opening pages recount a passage in the ministry of Buddha, the Hindu redeemer, cannot be more fitly closed than by the appeal ascribed by Ovid to Pythagoras, the Samian sage.

> Forbear, O mortals, to taint your bodies with forbidden food;
> Corn have we; the boughs bend under a load of fruit;
> Our vines abound in swelling grapes; our fields with wholesome herbs,
> Whereof those of a cruder kind may be softened and mellowed by fire.
> Nor is milk denied us, nor honey smelling of the fragrant thyme;
> Earth is lavish of her riches, and teems with kindly stores,
> Providing without slaughter or bloodshed for all manner of delights.
> The savage beasts indeed allay their hunger with flesh,
> But the wild horse, the flocks, the kine, subsist on grass:
> They only of a fierce and ravenous nature –
> Bears, wolves, Armenian tigers, and the angry brood of lions –
> These delight in meats reeking with the red tide of life.
> O impious custom, to bury entrails in entrails, to fatten a craving body with the flesh of its fellow,
> Maintaining the life of one creature by the murderous death of another!
> Is it possible indeed that amidst the plenty which earth, the best of parents, so bountifully bestows,
> Nothing can delight yon but to tear wounded flesh, and to renew the barbarous Cyclopean feasts?
> Cannot the desires of your ravenous and unrighteous appetite be appeased
> Save by the destruction of the life of your fellows?
> But they of ancient times, justly called the Age of Gold,
> Content with the fruit of their trees and the herbs of earth, stained not their lips with blood;
> Then might the birds in safety traverse the airy expanse and the hare move fearless over field and moor,
> Nor were even the credulous fish beguiled by the deceitful hook;

Snares and treachery were unknown, no dread of fraud disturbed the mind, all things were full of peace.

Then arose that impious contriver of innovations, who first envied man his innocent repasts,

(p. 120)

And, gorging his lustful appetite with flesh, opened a door for cruelty.

What I have you merited to die, O sheep! placid, inoffensive race, born to bless and serve us,

Whose full udders yield sweet milk, whose fleeces clothe us with soft raiment,

Comforting us more by your lives than by your deaths?

And you, O oxen! guileless and docile, mild and innocent, made to labour for man,

He indeed is unmindful of your services, and all unworthy the gifts of Ceres,

Who, having but now unyoked his gentle labourer from the plough, can harden himself to shed his blood!

To smite with an axe that neck worn in his service with toil, which so often has renewed his else unfruitful fields,

Bringing him so many a rich and welcome harvest

Nor is it enough that men commit such crimes as these,

They ascribe to the Gods their own wickedness, and pretend that even the Divine Powers' delight in innocent blood:

A victim without spot and of surpassing beauty – (as if to be perfect were to deserve death) –

Such an one, adorned with garlands and with gold, they lead to the votive altar;

He hears the prayer of the priest, not knowing what it means,

And sees the corn he helped to produce, laid between the horns on his forehead,

Then, struck by the sacrificial knife, he dyes with his lifeblood the blade

Whose gleam perchance he beheld in the transparent fountain at his feet.

Straightway the priest tears the entrails from his panting bosom,

Seeking to learn from these the mind of the high Gods!

Whence have men this lust for unlawful food?

How, O mortal race, can you endure to eat of it?

Refrain, I beseech you t give heed to my precepts!

And, when you would feast on the limbs of the dismembered ox,

Know and reflect that it is the tiller of your fields you would destroy!

How unholy a custom, how easy a way to human murder he makes for himself

Who cuts the innocent throat of the calf, and hears unmoved its mournful plaints!

And slaughters the little kid, whose cry is like the cry of a child,
Or devours the birds of the air which his own hands have fed!
Ah, how little is wanting to fill the cup of his wickedness!
What unrighteous deed is he not ready to commit!
Suffer the ox to plough, and impute his death to age and Nature's hand,
Let the sheep continue to yield us sheltering woo), and the goats the produce of their loaded udders,
Banish from among you nets and snares and painful artifices,
Conspire no longer against the birds, nor scare the meek deer, nor hide with fraud the crooked hook;
Make war on noxious creatures, and kill them only, But let your mouths be empty of blood, and satisfied with pure and natural repasts! *(1)*

FOOTNOTES

(121:1) *Metam*, lib. xv.

www.ingramcontent.com/pod-product-compliance
Lightning Source LLC
Chambersburg PA
CBHW020452220526
45464CB00002B/955